W9-BRF-319

Flat Belly Diet.®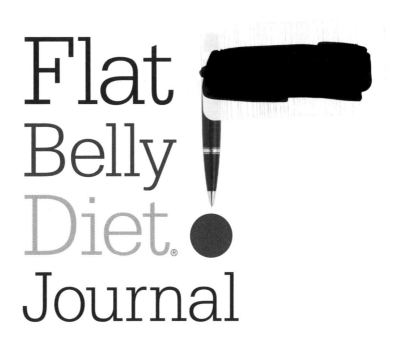
Journal

This book is intended as a reference volume only, not as a medical manual. The information presented here is designed to help you make informed decisions about your health. It is not intended as a substitute for any treatment that may have been prescribed by your doctor. If you suspect that you have a medical problem, we urge you to seek competent medical care.

Mention of specific companies, organizations, or authorities in this book does not imply endorsement by the author or publisher, nor does mention of specific companies, organizations, or authorities imply their endorsement of this book, its author, or the publisher. Internet addresses and telephone numbers were accurate at the time this book went to press.

© 2008 by Rodale Inc.

All rights reserved. No part of this publication may be reproduced or transmitted in any form or by any means, electronic or mechanical, including photocopying, recording, or any other information storage and retrieval system, without the written permission of the publisher.

Rodale books may be purchased for business or promotional use or for special sales. For information, please write to:
Special Markets Department, Rodale Inc., 733 Third Avenue, New York, NY 10017

Prevention is a registered trademark of Rodale Inc.
Flat Belly Diet is a registered trademark of Rodale Inc.

Printed in the United States of America
Rodale Inc. makes every effort to use acid-free ♾, recycled paper ♾.

Book design by Jill Armus

Library of Congress Cataloging-in-Publication Data is on file with the publisher.

ISBN-13: 978-1-60529-403-2
ISBN-10: 1-60529-403-9

2   4   6   8   10   9   7   5   3   1   paperback

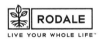

We inspire and enable people to improve their lives and the world around them
For more of our products visit **rodalestore.com** or call 800-848-4735

Flat Belly Diet! Journal

BY LIZ VACCARIELLO, Editor-in-Chief of **Prevention**.

RODALE

Introduction

THERE IS NO doubt in our minds that one single tool has the most powerful impact on long-term dietary change: a food diary. We admit that it's not the freshest or most cutting-edge advice, but you hear it over and over again because—well, it works!

A new Kaiser Permanente study involving more than 1,600 people (average age 55) in four cities (Portland, Oregon; Baltimore, Maryland; Durham, North Carolina; and Baton Rouge, Louisiana) found that those who kept a food journal seven days a week lost twice as much weight over six months compared to those who weren't regular recorders (18 pounds vs. 9).

Food diaries are like a nutritional checkbook. Without balancing your checkbook, it's nearly impossible to keep track of your finances, and the same is true for food. Most Americans overestimate how much they have to "spend" calorie-wise, underestimate how much they eat, and underestimate the number of calories in lots of foods. Most also overestimate the number of calories they burn when exercising. (Can you imagine accidentally spending more than you make month after month because you were off in your calculations? Yikes!)

But this goes beyond calories. Writing it all down dramatically raises your awareness and helps you to see the "big picture" of your relationship with food, including not just how much you eat but why, when, and how. You'll probably start seeing patterns you weren't aware of—patterns that may be holding you back from success. And until you know about and understand them, they're nearly impossible to change.

Cynthia Sass, MPH, RD, who created the diet, has had more than fifteen years of experience as a dietitian and food coach. Just about every client she's ever asked to keep a food journal has been downright surprised by what they've learned. Most thought they had a pretty good handle on their habits. They'd proclaim, "I always eat breakfast," "I eat tons of fruit and vegetables," or "I hardly ever snack," but after journaling, they'd find out that their perceptions were pretty far off.

If you're hesitant, keep in mind that the main goal of a food journal isn't to police yourself: It's to learn about yourself. Diaries aren't meant to make you feel ashamed or scolded. They just help you get to know—and get real with—yourself.

When we first launched the *Flat Belly Diet*, we offered readers the opportunity to track their meals online at flatbellydiet.com. While many people found that extremely helpful, others wanted a physical book to write in. So we decided to create this journal for you to help you make the most of the *Flat Belly Diet*. We hope you find it useful!

—Liz Vaccariello, Editor-in-Chief

The Four-Day Anti-Bloat Jumpstart

The Four-Day Anti-Bloat Jumpstart isn't just about beating bloat; it's also extremely important in sparking your emotional commitment to the entire program. The four-day plan includes a prescribed list of foods and drinks that will help flush out fluid, reduce water retention, and relieve digestive issues like gas and constipation, which can make your belly puff unnecessarily. You'll drink Sassy Water (a signature recipe developed by Cynthia) while eating healthy foods like fruits, vegetables, and whole grains.

The jumpstart abolishes the foods, beverages, and behaviors that cause your belly to pooch out. And—as a bonus—the plan provides guidelines for reducing the chances of ever feeling this way again. The Four-Day Anti-Bloat Jumpstart is carefully designed to deflate your tummy and spur your body to release excess fluid.

The following information describes the foods you'll eat and those you'll need to avoid during the four-day program, as well as some dos and don'ts. Keep in mind that we make it easy for you—all your meals are already planned.

WHAT TO DO
FOLLOW THE FOUR-DAY MEAL PLAN EXACTLY.

This includes four smaller meals, one of which is a refreshing, belly fat–blasting smoothie. You'll notice a few staples, including sunflower seeds, flaxseed oil, string cheese, and carrots. There are three reasons you'll see these items appear repeatedly. First, we tried to limit the amount of food you have to buy to get started—and ensure you'll eat it before it goes bad. Second, we wanted to deliver a lot of nutritional and bloat-free bang for the buck. Finally, we chose foods that need no added salt or condiments to taste good, so you won't be tempted to reach for one of these potential bloat-promoters.

EAT FOUR MEALS A DAY.

The Four-Day Jumpstart includes fewer calories—about 1,200 daily—than you'll be eating on the rest of the *Flat Belly Diet*, which allows about 1,600 per day. Eating less for these four days reduces the amount of food in your GI tract at any one time, cuts back on the release of stomach acids, and gets your body used to a four-meal-a-day schedule.

DRINK ONE FULL RECIPE OF SASSY WATER EVERY DAY.

The ingredients in Sassy Water aren't just for flavor: The ginger helps calm and soothe your GI tract. Even more important, the simple act of making this Sassy Water every day will serve as a reminder during the Jumpstart that life is a little bit different and that things are going to change.

SASSY WATER

2 liters water (about 8½ cups)
1 teaspoon freshly grated ginger root
1 medium cucumber, peeled and thinly sliced
1 medium lemon, thinly sliced
12 small spearmint leaves

Combine all ingredients in a large pitcher, chill in the refrigerator, and let flavors blend overnight. Drink the entire pitcher by the end of each day.

TAKE A QUICK 5-MINUTE AFTER-MEAL WALK.

Moving your body helps release air that has been trapped in your GI tract, relieving pressure and bloating.

EAT SLOWLY.

When you eat fast, you take in large gulps of air, which get trapped in your digestive system and cause bloating.

WORK YOUR MIND.

The first days of a diet are never easy, and these four days are no exception. I'm asking you to change how you eat and to give up some of the foods you're used to eating or drinking—and perhaps imagine you can't live without. Of course, it's going to be worth it in the end—it does work, and you will see your belly shrink. But until you see that poof disappear, you'll need a mental tune-up. That's where my Mind Tricks come in. Mind Tricks are a way of giving a meal importance—making it a special, you-focused moment. They'll help you stay mindful of what you're eating and why.

WHAT TO AVOID

The following foods are off-limits for the four days of the Jumpstart:

THE SALT SHAKER, SALT-BASED SEASONINGS, AND HIGHLY PROCESSED FOODS

Water is attracted to sodium, so when you take in higher-than-usual amounts of sodium, you'll temporarily retain more fluid—which contributes to a sluggish feeling, a puffy appearance, and extra water weight.

EXCESS CARBS

As a backup energy source, your muscles store a type of carbohydrate called glycogen. Every gram of glycogen is stored with about 3 grams of water. But unless you're running a marathon tomorrow, you don't need all this stockpiled fuel. Decreasing your carbohydrate intake temporarily can train your body to access this stored fuel and burn it off. At the same time, you'll be draining off all that excess stored fluid.

BULKY RAW FOODS

A half-cup serving of cooked carrots delivers the same nutrition as 1 cup raw, but it takes up less room in your GI tract. Eat only cooked vegetables, smaller portions of unsweetened dried fruit, and canned fruits in natural juice. This will allow you to meet your nutrient needs without expanding your GI tract with extra volume.

GASSY FOODS

Certain foods simply create more gas in your GI tract. They include legumes, cauliflower, broccoli, Brussels sprouts, cabbage, onions, peppers, and citrus fruits.

CHEWING GUM

You probably don't realize this, but when you chew gum, you swallow air. All that air gets trapped in your GI tract and causes pressure, bloating, and belly expansion.

SUGAR ALCOHOLS

These sugar substitutes, which go by the names xylitol or maltitol, are often found in low-calorie or low-carb products because they taste sweet. Like fiber, your GI tract can't absorb most of them. That's good for your calorie bottom line, but not so good for your belly. Sugar alcohols cause gas, abdominal distention, bloating, and diarrhea. Avoid them.

FRIED FOODS

Fatty foods, especially the fried variety, are digested more slowly, causing you to feel heavy and bloated.

SPICY FOODS

Foods seasoned with black pepper, nutmeg, cloves, chili powder, hot sauces, onions, garlic, mustard, chili, barbecue sauce, horseradish, ketchup, tomato sauce, or vinegar can all stimulate the release of stomach acid, which can cause irritation.

CARBONATED DRINKS

All those bubbles end up in your belly! Avoid these completely.

ALCOHOL, COFFEE, TEA, HOT COCOA, AND ACIDIC FRUIT JUICES

Each of these high-acidic beverages can irritate your GI tract, causing swelling.

In addition, try to avoid the Four Bad Guys of Bloat:

STRESS

It triggers a complex sequence of hormonal fluctuations that raise blood pressure and divert blood to your extremities, where energy is most needed. This process allows you to run faster or lift more if necessary, but it also causes your digestive system to slow down significantly. As a result, your last meal may stick around in your intestine, causing bloat.

LACK OF FLUID

You've probably heard you need about eight glasses of water a day. Drinking water and even eating "watery" foods like melon, greens, and other fruits and vegetables have enormous health benefits, including warding off fatigue, maintaining your body's proper fluid balance, and guarding against water retention and constipation, which can cause bloating. Eight glasses is just a guideline; everyone's fluid needs vary according to activity level and body type.

LACK OF SLEEP

Too little sleep disrupts the intricate workings of your nervous system, which controls the rhythmic contractions of your GI tract and helps keep things humming along. It also affects your overall ability to manage and cope with stress. It's important to get at least seven hours of sleep a night.

AIR TRAVEL

The average plane maintains cabin pressure equal to 5,000 to 8,000 feet above sea level in order to provide a comfortable atmosphere for the passengers. At that altitude, free air in the body cavities tends to expand by around 25 percent. Pressure changes also increase the production of gases in your GI tract. As the pressure in the cabin drops, the air in your intestines expands, causing bloating and discomfort. Your best defense is to drink as much water as possible before and during your flight and to walk around as often as possible.

Your Four-Day Shopping List

PRODUCE

- ❑ 2 pints grape tomatoes
- ❑ 1 pint fresh or frozen green beans
- ❑ 2 large red potatoes
- ❑ 10 oz bag baby carrots
- ❑ Half pint cremini mushrooms
- ❑ 1 large yellow squash
- ❑ 4 medium cucumbers
- ❑ 4 medium lemons

DAIRY

- ❑ ½ gallon lactose-free skim milk
- ❑ 1 package low-fat string cheese

FROZEN FOODS

- ❑ 10 oz bag frozen unsweetened blueberries
- ❑ 10 oz bag frozen unsweetened peaches
- ❑ 10 oz bag frozen unsweetened strawberries

DRY GOODS

- ❑ 12 oz box unsweetened corn flakes
- ❑ 12 oz box unsweetened puffed rice cereal
- ❑ 12 oz box instant Cream of Wheat®
- ❑ 14 oz box instant brown rice
- ❑ 24 oz jar unsweetened applesauce
- ❑ 8 oz can pineapple tidbits canned in pineapple juice

- ❑ 1 cup bulk (or 1 small package) roasted or raw unsalted sunflower seeds
- ❑ 8 oz bottle cold-pressed organic flaxseed oil
- ❑ 8 oz bottle olive oil
- ❑ 15 oz package raisins
- ❑ 7 oz container dried plums

SPICES

- ❑ 1–2 knuckles fresh ginger root
- ❑ 2 bunches fresh mint

MEAT/SEAFOOD

- ❑ 2 packages organic deli turkey
- ❑ ¼ pound tilapia
- ❑ ⅓ pound boneless skinless chicken breast
- ❑ ¼ pound turkey breast cutlet
- ❑ 3 oz can chunk light tuna in water

ANY OF THESE APPROVED SALT-FREE SEASONINGS

- ❑ Original and Italian medley Mrs. Dash® salt-free seasoning blends
- ❑ Fresh or dried: basil, bay leaf, cinnamon, curry powder, dill, ginger, lemon or lime juice, marjoram, mint, oregano, paprika, pepper, rosemary, sage, tarragon, or thyme
- ❑ Aged balsamic vinegar

THE FOUR-DAY ANTI-BLOAT MENU, DAY 1

DATE:

BREAKFAST

- ❏ 1 cup unsweetened cornflakes
- ❏ 1 cup skim milk
- ❏ ½ cup unsweetened applesauce
- ❏ ¼ cup roasted or raw unsalted sunflower seeds
- ❏ Glass of Sassy Water

MIND TRICK: Say hello, sunshine! Enjoy breakfast near a sunny window. Morning sunlight has been shown to be a mood booster and will set your body's master clock for maximum all-day energy.

LUNCH

- ❏ 4 oz organic deli turkey, rolled up
- ❏ 1 low-fat string cheese
- ❏ 1 pint fresh grape tomatoes
- ❏ Glass of Sassy Water

MIND TRICK: Put some color in your day. Before sitting down, arrange a few cut flowers in a vase and place it on the table. You're working hard on this diet. You deserve something special for your efforts.

SNACK

- ❏ Blueberry Smoothie: Blend 1 cup skim milk and 1 cup frozen unsweetened blueberries in blender for 1 minute. Transfer to glass and stir in 1 Tbsp cold-pressed organic flaxseed oil, or serve with 1 Tbsp sunflower or pumpkin seeds.

MIND TRICK: Take a virtual vacation. Put on some Hawaiian music while you're preparing your meal and transport yourself to a beach with lapping water and coconut palms. For good measure, rub a little suntan oil on your face and inhale deeply. It's snowing outside? Nah. You're in Hawaii.

DINNER

- ❏ 1 cup cooked green beans
- ❏ 4 oz grilled tilapia
- ❏ ½ cup roasted red potatoes drizzled with 1 tsp olive oil
- ❏ Glass of Sassy Water

MIND TRICK: Resize your settings. Set your table with smaller plates and bowls. It'll make you feel like you have more food than you actually do.

JOURNAL, DAY 1

DATE:

BREAKFAST

MOOD:

THOUGHTS/CHALLENGES:

HUNGER BEFORE:
-5 -3 0 3 5 7

HUNGER AFTER:
-5 -3 0 3 5 7

LUNCH

MOOD:

THOUGHTS/CHALLENGES:

HUNGER BEFORE:
-5 -3 0 3 5 7

HUNGER AFTER:
-5 -3 0 3 5 7

SNACK

MOOD:

THOUGHTS/CHALLENGES:

HUNGER BEFORE:
-5 -3 0 3 5 7

HUNGER AFTER:
-5 -3 0 3 5 7

DINNER

MOOD:

THOUGHTS/CHALLENGES:

HUNGER BEFORE:
-5 -3 0 3 5 7

HUNGER AFTER:
-5 -3 0 3 5 7

Hunger Rating

-5 = STARVING. You want to devour the first thing you see and have a hard time slowing down.

-3 = OVERLY HUNGRY AND IRRITABLE. You feel like you waited too long to eat.

0 = MILD TO MODERATE HUNGER. You may have physical symptoms of hunger, like a growling tummy and that "I need to eat soon" feeling, but you aren't starving or experiencing any unpleasant symptoms such as a headache or shaking.

3 = HUNGER BUT NOT CRAVING FREE. You're full, but you don't feel quite satisfied; your thoughts are still focused on food.

5 = JUST RIGHT. Your hunger is gone, and you feel satisfied. Your mind is off food, and you're ready to take on the next task. You feel energized.

7 = A LITTLE TOO MUCH. You think you overdid it. Your tummy feels stretched and uncomfortable. You feel kind of sluggish.

THE FOUR-DAY ANTI-BLOAT MENU, DAY 2

DATE:

BREAKFAST

- ☐ 1 cup unsweetened puffed rice cereal
- ☐ 1 cup skim milk
- ☐ ¼ cup roasted or raw unsalted sunflower seeds
- ☐ 4 oz pineapple tidbits canned in juice
- ☐ Glass of Sassy Water

MIND TRICK: Find a one-meal-only mantra. Pick a calming word or phrase, such as "I'm doing this diet for me." Repeat it after every bite.

LUNCH

- ☐ 3 oz chunk light tuna in water
- ☐ 1 cup steamed baby carrots
- ☐ 1 low-fat string cheese
- ☐ Glass of Sassy Water

MIND TRICK: Convert a friend. Invite a pal to have lunch with you today and explain your meal. Try to remember as many principles of the Jumpstart as possible. This will help you remember why you're doing this, even though it's such a departure from your normal routine.

SNACK

- ☐ Pineapple Smoothie: Blend 1 cup skim milk, 4 oz canned pineapple tidbits in juice, and a handful of ice in blender for 1 minute. Transfer to glass and stir in 1 Tbsp cold-pressed organic flaxseed oil, or serve with 1 Tbsp sunflower or pumpkin seeds.

MIND TRICK: Hang up some inspiration. Keep, say, your "skinny jeans" on a hanger in full view, so you pass them every day. They'll serve as a reminder of your ultimate weight loss goal. They *will* fit you again.

DINNER

- ☐ 1 cup fresh cremini mushrooms sautéed with 1 tsp olive oil
- ☐ 3 oz grilled chicken breast
- ☐ ½ cup cooked brown rice
- ☐ Glass of Sassy Water

MIND TRICK: Sing while you prepare dinner. According to German researchers, you can enjoy up to a 240 percent immunity boost as well as an increase of anti-stress hormones simply by singing.

JOURNAL, DAY 2

DATE:

BREAKFAST	
MOOD:	THOUGHTS/CHALLENGES:

HUNGER BEFORE:
-5 -3 0 3 5 7

HUNGER AFTER:
-5 -3 0 3 5 7

LUNCH	
MOOD:	THOUGHTS/CHALLENGES:

HUNGER BEFORE:
-5 -3 0 3 5 7

HUNGER AFTER:
-5 -3 0 3 5 7

SNACK	
MOOD:	THOUGHTS/CHALLENGES:

HUNGER BEFORE:
-5 -3 0 3 5 7

HUNGER AFTER:
-5 -3 0 3 5 7

DINNER	
MOOD:	THOUGHTS/CHALLENGES:

HUNGER BEFORE:
-5 -3 0 3 5 7

HUNGER AFTER:
-5 -3 0 3 5 7

Hunger Rating

–5 = STARVING. You want to devour the first thing you see and have a hard time slowing down.

–3 = OVERLY HUNGRY AND IRRITABLE. You feel like you waited too long to eat.

0 = MILD TO MODERATE HUNGER. You may have physical symptoms of hunger, like a growling tummy and that "I need to eat soon" feeling, but you aren't starving or experiencing any unpleasant symptoms such as a headache or shaking.

3 = HUNGER BUT NOT CRAVING FREE. You're full, but you don't feel quite satisfied; your thoughts are still focused on food.

5 = JUST RIGHT. Your hunger is gone, and you feel satisfied. Your mind is off food, and you're ready to take on the next task. You feel energized.

7 = A LITTLE TOO MUCH. You think you overdid it. Your tummy feels stretched and uncomfortable. You feel kind of sluggish.

THE FOUR-DAY ANTI-BLOAT MENU, DAY 3

DATE:

BREAKFAST	
❑ 1 cup unsweetened cornflakes ❑ 1 cup skim milk ❑ ¼ cup roasted or raw unsalted sunflower seeds ❑ 2 Tbsp raisins ❑ Glass of Sassy Water	**MIND TRICK:** Focus on your moment. This morning, eat your breakfast with no distraction—no radio, no morning show, no newspaper. Focus on the flavor of each bite.

LUNCH	
❑ 4 oz organic deli turkey, rolled up ❑ 1 low-fat string cheese ❑ 1 pint grape tomatoes ❑ Glass of Sassy Water	**MIND TRICK:** Bring in some bling. Serve your Sassy Water in the finest crystal glass you own. Make this your Flat Belly glass, and use it at every meal.

SNACK	
❑ Peach Smoothie: Blend 1 cup skim milk and 1 cup frozen unsweetened peaches in blender for 1 minute. Transfer to glass and stir in 1 Tbsp cold-pressed organic flaxseed oil, or serve with 1 Tbsp sunflower or pumpkin seeds.	**MIND TRICK:** Give thanks. Take a moment of gratitude for the food you are eating, the body you are nurturing, and the life you're enhancing. No need to get religious—it's perfectly okay to thank the peach farmer and your parents!

DINNER	
❑ 1 cup cooked green beans ❑ 3 oz grilled or baked turkey breast cutlet ❑ ½ cup roasted red potatoes drizzled with 1 tsp olive oil ❑ Glass of Sassy Water	**MIND TRICK:** Think about yourself. As you eat this meal, reflect on all you're doing to care for your body and your spirit.

JOURNAL, DAY 3

DATE:

BREAKFAST

MOOD:

THOUGHTS/CHALLENGES:

HUNGER BEFORE:
-5 -3 0 3 5 7

HUNGER AFTER:
-5 -3 0 3 5 7

LUNCH

MOOD:

THOUGHTS/CHALLENGES:

HUNGER BEFORE:
-5 -3 0 3 5 7

HUNGER AFTER:
-5 -3 0 3 5 7

SNACK

MOOD:

THOUGHTS/CHALLENGES:

HUNGER BEFORE:
-5 -3 0 3 5 7

HUNGER AFTER:
-5 -3 0 3 5 7

DINNER

MOOD:

THOUGHTS/CHALLENGES:

HUNGER BEFORE:
-5 -3 0 3 5 7

HUNGER AFTER:
-5 -3 0 3 5 7

Hunger Rating

–5 = STARVING. You want to devour the first thing you see and have a hard time slowing down.

–3 = OVERLY HUNGRY AND IRRITABLE. You feel like you waited too long to eat.

0 = MILD TO MODERATE HUNGER. You may have physical symptoms of hunger, like a growling tummy and that "I need to eat soon" feeling, but you aren't starving or experiencing any unpleasant symptoms such as a headache or shaking.

3 = HUNGER BUT NOT CRAVING FREE. You're full, but you don't feel quite satisfied; your thoughts are still focused on food.

5 = JUST RIGHT. Your hunger is gone, and you feel satisfied. Your mind is off food, and you're ready to take on the next task. You feel energized.

7 = A LITTLE TOO MUCH. You think you overdid it. Your tummy feels stretched and uncomfortable. You feel kind of sluggish.

THE FOUR-DAY ANTI-BLOAT MENU, DAY 4

DATE:

BREAKFAST

- ❏ 1 packet instant Cream of Wheat®
- ❏ 1 cup skim milk
- ❏ ¼ cup roasted or raw unsalted sunflower seeds
- ❏ 2 dried plums
- ❏ Glass of Sassy Water

MIND TRICK: Laugh it up. A 4-year-old laughs around 400 times a day; an adult, around 15. Today, even if you're alone when you sit down to your meal, laugh at your bowl of Cream of Wheat, and howl at your glass of Sassy Water.

LUNCH

- ❏ 4 oz organic deli turkey, rolled up
- ❏ 1 cup steamed baby carrots
- ❏ 1 low-fat string cheese
- ❏ Glass of Sassy Water

MIND TRICK: Arrange your plate. Take a few minutes to prepare today's lunch with the flair of a gourmet chef. Wrap the turkey slices around the cheese and carrots, then slice on the bias and arrange. Garnish with a few sprigs of fresh herbs.

SNACK

- ❏ Strawberry Smoothie: Blend 1 cup skim milk and 1 cup frozen unsweetened strawberries in blender for 1 minute. Transfer to glass and stir in 1 Tbsp cold-pressed organic flaxseed oil, or serve with 1 Tbsp sunflower or pumpkin seeds.

MIND TRICK: Before you sit down to eat, close your eyes and say something kind and reassuring about your body. Mention how much you love your arms or how people tell you you have great eyes or a fantastic smile.

DINNER

- ❏ 1 cup yellow squash sautéed with 1 tsp olive oil
- ❏ 3 oz grilled chicken breast
- ❏ ½ cup cooked brown rice
- ❏ Glass of Sassy Water

MIND TRICK: Serve today's dinner on your best china. Set a proper place setting with the good silver and the damask napkins.

JOURNAL, DAY 4

DATE:

BREAKFAST	
MOOD:	THOUGHTS/CHALLENGES:
HUNGER BEFORE: -5 -3 0 3 5 7	HUNGER AFTER: -5 -3 0 3 5 7

LUNCH	
MOOD:	THOUGHTS/CHALLENGES:
HUNGER BEFORE: -5 -3 0 3 5 7	HUNGER AFTER: -5 -3 0 3 5 7

SNACK	
MOOD:	THOUGHTS/CHALLENGES:
HUNGER BEFORE: -5 -3 0 3 5 7	HUNGER AFTER: -5 -3 0 3 5 7

DINNER	
MOOD:	THOUGHTS/CHALLENGES:
HUNGER BEFORE: -5 -3 0 3 5 7	HUNGER AFTER: -5 -3 0 3 5 7

Hunger Rating

–5 = STARVING. You want to devour the first thing you see and have a hard time slowing down.

–3 = OVERLY HUNGRY AND IRRITABLE. You feel like you waited too long to eat.

0 = MILD TO MODERATE HUNGER. You may have physical symptoms of hunger, like a growling tummy and that "I need to eat soon" feeling, but you aren't starving or experiencing any unpleasant symptoms such as a headache or shaking.

3 = HUNGER BUT NOT CRAVING FREE. You're full, but you don't feel quite satisfied; your thoughts are still focused on food.

5 = JUST RIGHT. Your hunger is gone, and you feel satisfied. Your mind is off food, and you're ready to take on the next task. You feel energized.

7 = A LITTLE TOO MUCH. You think you overdid it. Your tummy feels stretched and uncomfortable. You feel kind of sluggish.

Three Rules to Eat By

Once you've completed the Jumpstart, you'll see a flatter belly and feel the jolt of confidence that comes with achieving such speedy results. Continued success—losing belly fat, that is—is a sure thing if you follow the three simple *Flat Belly Diet* rules.

RULE #1: **Eat a MUFA at every meal.** Make this your mantra. Unlike a Saturday-morning doughnut splurge that leaves you feeling sacked out and groggy for the rest of the day, MUFA foods, when eaten in the right amounts, have an amazing ability to provide steady, even fuel and quell the appetite. When enjoyed with complex carbohydrates, MUFA foods help slow digestion, which is one of the ways they help control blood sugar and insulin levels, as well as manage hunger. If you

Are You Really Hungry?

The line between emotional eating and true hunger is actually quite clear. Researchers from the University of Texas Counseling and Mental Health Center have identified five ways to tell the difference between the two. Recognizing these signals can help you distinguish an emotional need for food from a physical one.

1. Emotional hunger comes on suddenly, while physical hunger is gradual.
2. You feel physical hunger below the neck with a grumbling stomach. Emotional hunger happens in your head, as in a craving for ice cream.
3. When only a certain food will meet your need—only a slice of pizza or chocolate will do—your hunger is emotional. When you body truly requires fuel, you're more open to other food options.
4. Emotional hunger aches to be satisfied immediately. Physical hunger can wait.
5. Emotional hunger, when acted upon, leaves you feeling guilty. Physical hunger doesn't.

The next time a craving strikes, try this: Tune out the signals coming from the neck up. Are you physically hungry? Ask yourself what you're feeling emotionally and how you can meet these mental (vs. physical) needs.

eat fruit and yogurt alone and have your MUFA a few hours later, it won't have the same satiating effect of enjoying the three foods together. That said, it's also important to get a range of MUFAs every day. I know you might have been hoping that you'd finally found the one magic diet that requires eating chocolate four times a day, but the reality here is that the easiest way to enjoy a healthy diet is to make sure it's varied. So mix up those MUFAs!

If you want to replace a MUFA in a particular recipe with another, just make sure they each have roughly the same number of calories. Consult the list on page 30 for suggestions.

RULE #2: **Stick to 400 calories per meal.** The *Flat Belly Diet* is a 1,600-calorie plan. We chose this number because this daily allowance is what it takes for a 40-plus-year-old woman of average height, frame size, and activity level to achieve and maintain ideal body weight—without unnecessary and unhealthy compromises in terms of enjoyment, energy, and overall well-being, not to mention bone density and muscle mass. Dividing your 1,600 calories evenly over three meals plus a substantial snack steadily fuels your energy and metabolism. That means you keep feeling good and burning fat all day long.

RULE #3: **Never go more than 4 hours without eating.** Timing is vital to making the most of the appetite-quelling and belly-fat-burning powers of your MUFAs. Eating smaller MUFA-rich meals more often rather than two or three larger meals spread out farther keeps your blood sugar stable, which fends off cravings and prevents fluctuations in insulin that signal your body to store fat. It also keeps your energy up and your hunger at bay, so you don't have bouts of fatigue and a grumbling tummy to contend with between meals—and the irritable disposition that comes with being tired and underfed.

These rules work in tandem to form the basic structure of the *Flat Belly Diet*. It is the combination of MUFAs at every meal *plus* the reduced but reasonable calorie guideline *plus* the frequency of whole-some meals that enables your body to stay energized and healthy while unloading belly fat.

WHAT'S A MUFA?

As you know, "MUFA" (MOO-fah) stands for "monounsaturated fatty acid," a type of heart-healthy, disease-fighting, "good" fat found in foods like almonds, peanut butter, olive oil, avocados, and even chocolate. MUFAs are an unsaturated fat and have the exact opposite effect of the unhealthy saturated and trans fats you've heard about in the news.

But there's more! MUFAs are delicious in and of themselves. Who doesn't love drizzling olive oil over a salad or grabbing a handful of chocolate chips? You'll find MUFA-rich foods incorporated into all the meal plans and Snack Packs. You can substitute one MUFA for another as long as the calorie counts are nearly equivalent. To get better acquainted with the five MUFA groups and learn how to buy, store, and prepare them, turn to page 25.

MAKING THE FLAT BELLY DIET WORK FOR YOU

In the *Flat Belly Diet!* and the *Flat Belly Diet! Cookbook*, we provided a wealth of quick and delicious recipes based on these three rules. But it's also easy to create your own *Flat Belly* meals. For each one, start by picking your MUFA and determining how many calories are left to work with. The basic components for any meal are MUFAs, lean proteins, whole grains or fruit, and (for lunch and dinner) vegetables. Visual cues are provided in parentheses. Here's how to build a *Flat Belly Diet* meal.

If your MUFA choice is nuts, seeds, or oil, add the following:

- 3 ounces lean protein (about the size of a deck of cards)
- 2 cups raw or steamed veggies (2 baseballs)

Dining out Flat Belly Style

Being on the *Flat Belly Diet* doesn't mean you never get a break from cooking for yourself. Here are a few key tips for staying on track when dining out.

1. Go online to look at the restaurant menu and find meals that resemble those in the book or your meal plans. If the restaurant doesn't have a Web site, call and ask about the menu or have a copy faxed to you.

2. Rely on a safe bet. You can always order a salad made of leafy greens and raw veggies (about the size of two baseballs) topped with grilled chicken or salmon (no more than a card-deck-size portion) with balsamic or red wine vinegar, and add 2 tablespoons (two thumb tips, from where your thumb bends to its top) of seeds or chopped nuts (bring them along) or 1 tablespoon olive oil. Add a computer-mouse-size serving of one of the following: whole grain roll; baked or roasted red, white, or sweet potato; brown or wild rice or a starchy veggie such as beans, peas, or corn. This meal should keep you within your calorie budget, and it contains a MUFA!

3. Or follow the guidelines for building your own Flat Belly meal (see the instructions below and to the left.)

- ½ cup cooked whole grain, such as brown or wild rice (about the size of a mini fruit cup) *or* 1 whole grain bread serving (such as half of a whole wheat pita) *or* 1 cup fruit (baseball)

  Example: 2 cups baby greens topped with 3 ounces grilled chicken, 2 tablespoons almonds, and 1 cup sliced apples

If your MUFA is avocado or olives, pair it with:

- 3 ounces lean protein *or* 2 ounces lean protein plus 1 dairy (such as 1 slice cheese or ¼ cup shredded or crumbled cheese)

- 2 cups raw or steamed veggies

- 1 cup starchy vegetables (beans, corn, peas, potatoes) *or* 1 cup cooked whole grain (such as brown or wild rice) *or* 2 whole grain bread servings (such as a full whole wheat pita, wrap, or English muffin)

Example: 3 ounces light water-packed tuna on top of 2 cups field greens topped with ½ cup garbanzo beans, ½ cup peas, and ¼ cup avocado

If your MUFA is dark chocolate, pair it with:

- 1 cup fruit plus 1 cup dairy such as fat-free milk, yogurt, or cottage cheese *or* whole grain such as 1 cup oatmeal or 1 whole grain waffle

  Example: ¼ cup chocolate chips mixed with 1 cup berries and 1 cup fat-free vanilla yogurt

What about Alcohol?

Whether or not you drink on the *Flat Belly Diet* is up to you. Current dietary guidelines recommend that if you don't drink, you should not start. In moderation, alcohol has been shown to lower the risk of heart disease, but it also carries risks. Just one drink a day is linked to an increased risk of breast cancer, and more-than-moderate drinking is tied to liver cirrhosis, high blood pressure, cancers of the upper gastrointestinal tract, stroke, injuries, and violence.

Some people are advised not to consume alcoholic beverages at all, including pregnant and lactating women and individuals taking medications that can interact with alcohol.

That said, most adults do consume alcohol, so if you do already drink, practice moderation, meaning one drink per day for women and up to two drinks per day for men. (One drink equals 12 ounces of regular beer, 5 ounces of wine, or 1.5 ounces—one shot—of 80-proof distilled spirits.) Each of these contains about 100 calories, so to stay on track with the *Flat Belly Diet*, you'll need to balance out those calories somehow. You can either burn 100 extra calories by exercising or shave 25 calories from each of your four meals—or 50 from two. Taking 100 calories out of a single 400-calorie meal can leave you feeling too hungry, and since alcohol is an appetite stimulant, that could be a recipe for overeating.

1. Oils

ANOINT YOUR MEALS with the most versatile MUFAs in the kitchen. Choose your oil based on use—cooking or drizzling—and flavor—strong or mild. HOW TO BUY AND USE: We recommend expeller pressed oils, a chemical-free extraction process. This natural method allows the oil to retain its natural color, aroma, and nutrients. Cold-pressed oil is expeller pressed in a heat-controlled environment to keep temperatures below 120°F. This is important for delicate oils like flaxseed. HOW TO STORE: Choose a container that holds only what you'll use within 2 months. As each container empties, it fills with oxygen, which causes the oil to oxidize, or deteriorate. This eventually creates a stale or bitter taste (like wet cardboard) and contributes to a breakdown of vitamin E and those precious MUFAs. Opt for dark glass jars or tins (rather than clear plastic bottles) to protect the oil from light, another source of flavor-sapping oxidation. You can store opened bottles of olive, canola, and peanut oils in a dark, cool place, such as the back of your pantry, but flaxseed oil should always be kept in the refrigerator because it breaks down more quickly at warmer temperatures.

HISTORY

Oils extracted from plant foods have been used in nearly every culture around the globe since ancient times. A 4,000-year-old kitchen unearthed by an archaeologist in Indiana revealed that large slabs of rock had been used to crush nuts, then extract the oil.

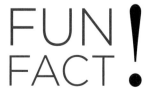

FUN FACT

SAFFLOWER OIL LABELED "HIGH-OLEIC" CONTAINS THE MOST BENEFICIAL MUFAS, FOLLOWED BY OLIVE OIL, AND THEN CANOLA OIL.

2. Olives

THERE'S AN OLIVE out there just for you. Choose your color (black or green) and pick your flavor (salty, sweet, or spicy). When you're all olived out, switch to tapenade, a deliciously pungent spread made from the crushed fruit.

HOW TO BUY AND USE: Fresh olives are available during the summer in specialty markets, but don't be lured unless you're a serious gourmet; they're incredibly bitter and inedible, thanks to a naturally occurring compound called oleuropin. Instead, choose the more appetizing olives at deli counters, which are sometimes pasteurized and cured in either oil, salt, or brine, and flavored with herbs or hot chilies. Olives can be purchased in jars and cans, as well as in bulk.

HOW TO STORE: Olives should be stored in the refrigerator after opening, either in the jar or an airtight container. If you bought your olives in cans, transfer any leftover into another airtight container before storing in the fridge.

HISTORY

Native to coastal regions of the Mediterranean, Asia, and areas of Africa, olives have been cultivated since 6000 BC and are one of the oldest known foods. These gems were brought to America by Spanish and Portuguese explorers during the 15th and 16th centuries and to California missions in the late 18th century. Today, most commercial olives are grown in Spain, Italy, Greece, and Turkey.

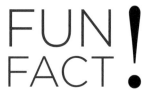

FUN FACT !

TRADITIONAL CHINESE MEDICINE USES OLIVE SOUP AS A SORE-THROAT RECIPE—THE ONLY OCCURRENCE OF THE OLIVE IN CHINESE CUISINE.

3. Nuts and Seeds

THESE MUFAS HAVE long been revered for their high levels of protein, fiber, and antioxidants (not to mention those healthy fats!). Sprinkle on yogurt, cereal, and salads; use as a topping for fish and chicken; or just snack on them out of hand.

HOW TO BUY AND USE: Nuts and seeds are sold in a variety of ways, including vacuum-sealed cans, glass jars, sealed bags, and in bulk. They can be whole, sliced, or chopped; raw or roasted; in or out of the shell. If purchasing in bulk, select a market that has high turnover and uses covered bins so they'll be perfectly fresh. Unshelled nuts should be free from cracks or holes, feel somewhat heavy for their size, and not rattle in the shell. Shelled nuts should be plump and look uniform in size and shape.

HOW TO STORE: Due to their high fat content, nuts and seeds tend to go rancid quickly once their shells are removed, especially if they're exposed to heat, light, and humidity during storage, so buy them as fresh as possible. When kept in a cool, dry place in an airtight container, raw, unshelled nuts will keep from 6 months to a year, while shelled nuts will stay fresh for 3 to 4 months under the same conditions. Shelled nuts can be stored for 4 months in a refrigerator and 6 months in a freezer.

HISTORY

Nuts and seeds have a long, extensive history. Almonds were prized by Egypt's pharaohs. The use of flaxseed goes as far back as the Stone Age and ancient Greece. Native Americans have been using sunflower seeds for more than 5,000 years, and peanuts were a staple of the Aztec diet.

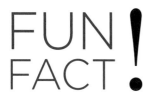

FUN FACT !

MACADAMIA NUTS PROVIDE MORE MUFA THAN ANY OTHER NUT OR SEED.

4. Avocados

ONCE A LUXURY FOOD reserved for royalty, supercreamy avocado is a feast of riches. Delicious mashed into a dip or sliced onto a salad, this MUFA is like butter, only better.

HOW TO BUY AND USE: When selecting any avocado, look for a fruit with slightly soft skin that yields slightly when you press it with your thumb. Avoid bruised, cracked, or indented fruit. Those with teardrop-shaped necks have usually been tree ripened and will have a richer taste than rounded specimens.

HISTORY

Avocados have been cultivated in South and Central America since 8000 BC. They were not introduced to the United States until the early 20th century, when they were first planted in California and Florida.

Once it's ripe, use a sharp knife to slice it lengthwise, guiding the knife gently around the pit. Then twist the two halves against each other in opposite directions to separate. The pit will still be lodged in one half. Carefully nudge the knife into the pit and twist it out to discard. You can either gently peel away the skin or carefully score the avocado while still in the peel, cutting into long slices or chunks, and use a spoon to separate it from the skin.

HOW TO STORE: A whole, ripe avocado with the skin on will keep in the refrigerator for a day or two. A slightly unripe avocado can be ripened in just a day or two by storing it in a paper bag and keeping it on the counter. To prevent a leftover portion from browning, coat the exposed flesh with lemon juice, wrap tightly in plastic wrap, and store in the refrigerator.

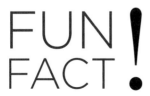

FUN FACT !

HASS AVOCADOS HAVE A MUCH CREAMIER CONSISTENCY THAN THEIR FLORIDA COUNTERPARTS AND PROVIDE ALMOST TWICE THE MUFA PER QUARTER-CUP SERVING.

5. Dark Chocolate

OUR MOST BELOVED MUFA. The one that makes us swoon. The one that makes every meal or snack a little bit sweeter. And the one that makes everyone want to start the *Flat Belly Diet*—and never stop.

HOW TO BUY AND USE: Semisweet and other dark chocolates are low enough in sugar and high enough in monounsaturated fats to get the MUFA

HISTORY

You're not the only one who loves chocolate. The ancient Mayans and Aztecs touted it as a food of the gods— and it's been a culinary mainstay ever since.

accolade in our book. Chocolates with a higher "cacao," or cocoa, content—the package usually lists the percentage—are typically darker, less sweet, and slightly more bitter, but in a good way. If you're used to milk chocolate, go dark gradually so you train your tastebuds to appreciate the stronger flavor of real, dark chocolate. You can buy chocolate in large chunks (popular with the baking set), as molded bars, or in chip form. I like chips because they're so easy to measure and use. (And when I want chocolate, I don't want to hassle with a knife and a grater!)

HOW TO STORE: Keep dark chocolate that's in its original sealed package in a cool dry area (60 to 75°F). Once opened, chocolate should be transferred to an airtight container or bag and stashed in the fridge (good) or freezer (best). During prolonged storage, chocolate will often "bloom," or develop a white blush. It's perfectly safe to eat, though not very appetizing to look at. One solution: Melt it—the bloom will disappear.

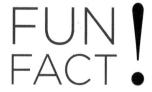

FUN FACT !

CHOCOLATE REALLY DOES MELT IN YOUR MOUTH BECAUSE ITS MELTING POINT IS SLIGHTLY BELOW HUMAN BODY TEMPERATURE.

YOUR MUFA SERVING CHART

FOOD	SERVING	CALORIES
SOYBEANS (EDAMAME), SHELLED AND BOILED	1 cup	298
SEMISWEET CHOCOLATE CHIPS	¼ cup	207
ALMOND BUTTER	2 Tbsp	200
CASHEW BUTTER	2 Tbsp	190
SUNFLOWER SEED BUTTER	2 Tbsp	190
NATURAL PEANUT BUTTER, CRUNCHY	2 Tbsp	188
NATURAL PEANUT BUTTER, SMOOTH	2 Tbsp	188
TAHINI (SESAME SEED PASTE)	2 Tbsp	178
PUMPKIN SEEDS	2 Tbsp	148
CANOLA OIL	1 Tbsp	124
FLAXSEED OIL (COLD-PRESSED ORGANIC)	1 Tbsp	120
MACADAMIA NUTS	2 Tbsp	120
SAFFLOWER OIL (HIGH OLEIC)	1 Tbsp	120
SESAME OR SOYBEAN OIL	1 Tbsp	120
SUNFLOWER OIL (HIGH OLEIC)	1 Tbsp	120
WALNUT OIL	1 Tbsp	120
OLIVE OIL	1 Tbsp	119
PEANUT OIL	1 Tbsp	119
PINE NUTS	2 Tbsp	113
BRAZIL NUTS	2 Tbsp	110
HAZELNUTS	2 Tbsp	110
PEANUTS	2 Tbsp	110
ALMONDS	2 Tbsp	109
CASHEWS	2 Tbsp	100
AVOCADO, CALIFORNIA (HASS)	¼ cup	96
PECANS	2 Tbsp	90
SUNFLOWER SEEDS	2 Tbsp	90
BLACK OLIVE TAPENADE	2 Tbsp	88
PISTACHIOS	2 Tbsp	88
WALNUTS	2 Tbsp	82
PESTO SAUCE	1 Tbsp	80
AVOCADO, FLORIDA	¼ cup	69
GREEN OLIVE TAPENADE	2 Tbsp	54
GREEN OR BLACK OLIVES	10 large	50

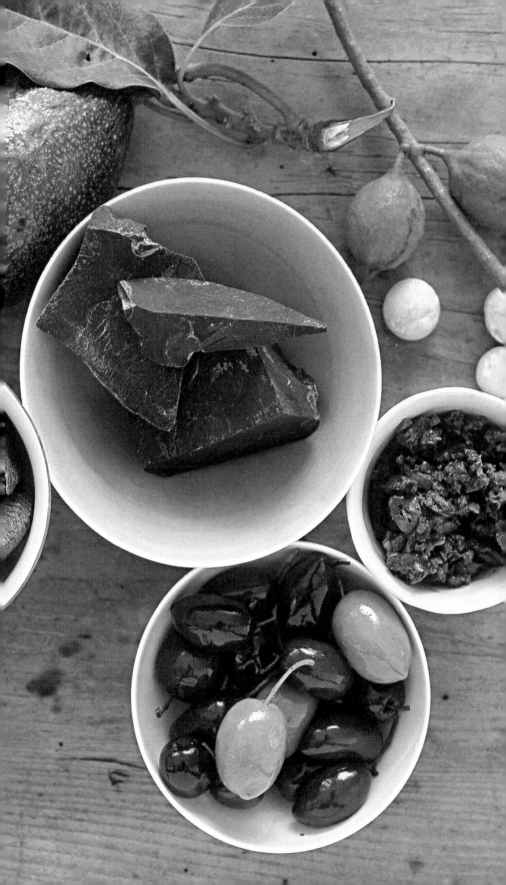

The Flat Belly Workout Basics

You'll lose weight on the Flat Belly Diet whether or not you exercise, but exercise will help you lose more faster. The Flat Belly Workout is built around three main components:

- Cardio exercise to burn calories and shed fat
- Strength training with weights to build muscle and boost metabolism
- Core-focused exercises to tone and tighten your midsection

CARDIO EXERCISE: FAT BLAST AND CALORIE TORCH WALKS

Cardio exercise burns calories, which is the only way to shrink the layer of fat covering your tummy muscles. Unless you're shedding that fat, you can spend hours doing ab exercises without seeing a change. We recommend walking for aerobic exercise because it's easy and accessible, but you can do anything you like: cycling, swimming, jogging, or using machines like treadmills, stair climbers, and elliptical trainers.

We recommend two types of cardio walks: **Fat Blast** and **Calorie Torch Walks**. Fat Blast walks are steadily paced walks guaranteed to burn off belly fat. You'll want to maintain an intensity of 5–6 (on a scale from 1–10), which should feel easy enough that you can talk freely but not sing. The length of these walks will increase each week, and as you become more fit, you should be able to walk at a faster pace.

Calorie Torch walks are set up to be executed in intervals, meaning periodic bursts of fast-paced walking (at a 7–8 intensity level, when you can talk in brief phrases but you'd rather not) interspersed with a moderate pace (at a 5–6 intensity level, when you can talk but not sing).

As you'll see on pages 34–35, we recommend that you do a cardio workout six days a week. If you can't fit in all six every week, don't beat yourself up: Just do what you can.

STRENGTH TRAINING: THE METABOLISM BOOST

The **Metabolism Boost** workout includes four combo moves that target multiple body parts—like your arms and legs—simultaneously. Each of these moves also has a balance challenge, so while you're working your arms, legs, butt, chest, and back, your core will be constantly engaged.

The four moves of the Metabolism Boost are:

- Lunge Press
- Side Lunge & Raise
- Squat Curl
- Pushup Row

CORE-FOCUSED EXERCISES: THE BELLY ROUTINE

The **Belly Routine** is nothing less than the best and most effective crunch-free exercise routine ever devised.

The five moves of the Belly Routine are:

- Bicycle
- Hover
- Roll-Up
- Arm & Leg Extension
- Ab Pike

As you'll see on pages 34–35, we recommend that you do three strength-training workouts and three core-strengthening workouts weekly, alternating between the Metabolism Boost and the Belly Routine. But if that's not possible, even one or two of each of these routines a week will help to speed up your results. If you do all six workouts one week, make sure to take one rest day each week. It doesn't matter what day you choose; feel free to work it around your schedule.

PUTTING IT ALL TOGETHER: YOUR 28-DAY FLAT BELLY WORKOUT PLAN

WEEK	DAY 1	DAY 2	DAY 3
1	Fat Blast Walk 30 min	Calorie Torch Walk 25 min	Fat Blast Walk 30 min
	The Belly Routine 10 reps	The Metabolism Boost 10 reps	The Belly Routine 10 reps
2	Fat Blast Walk 45 min	Calorie Torch Walk 35 min	Fat Blast Walk 45 min
	The Belly Routine 15 reps	The Metabolism Boost 15 reps	The Belly Routine 15 reps
3	Fat Blast Walk 60 min	Calorie Torch Walk 45 min	Fat Blast Walk 60 min
	The Belly Routine 2 sets, 10 reps	The Metabolism Boost 2 sets, 10 reps	The Belly Routine 2 sets, 10 reps
4	Fat Blast Walk 60 min	Calorie Torch Walk 45 min	Fat Blast Walk 60 min
	The Belly Routine 2 sets, 15 reps	The Metabolism Boost 2 sets, 15 reps	The Belly Routine 2 sets, 15 reps

DAY 4	DAY 5	DAY 6	DAY 7
Calorie Torch Walk 25 min	Fat Blast Walk 30 min	Calorie Torch Walk 25 min	REST
The Metabolism Boost 10 reps	The Belly Routine 10 reps	The Metabolism Boost 10 reps	
Calorie Torch Walk 35 min	Fat Blast Walk 45 min	Calorie Torch Walk 35 min	REST
The Metabolism Boost 15 reps	The Belly Routine 15 reps	The Metabolism Boost 15 reps	
Calorie Torch Walk 45 min	Fat Blast Walk 60 min	Calorie Torch Walk 45 min	REST
The Metabolism Boost 2 sets, 10 reps	The Belly Routine 2 sets, 10 reps	The Metabolism Boost 2 sets, 10 reps	
Calorie Torch Walk 45 min	Fat Blast Walk 60 min	Calorie Torch Walk 45 min	REST
The Metabolism Boost 2 sets, 15 reps	The Belly Routine 2 sets, 15 reps	The Metabolism Boost 2 sets, 15 reps	

The Joys of Journaling

As you know, keeping a food journal is an excellent way to help you focus on your new way of eating. Research has continually shown that keeping a log of what you eat and how you feel while you're eating really does help people stay on track with different lifestyle choices. In addition to being good for the soul, there is now increasing evidence to support the concept that journaling has a positive impact on physical well-being.

University of Texas at Austin researcher James Pennebaker, PhD, has scientifically shown that regular journaling strengthens immune cells, called T-lymphocytes. Other research indicates that journaling decreases the symptoms of asthma and rheumatoid arthritis. Pennebaker believes that writing about stressful events helps you come to terms with them, thus reducing the impact of these stressors on your physical health.

HOW TO USE THIS JOURNAL

Your *Flat Belly Diet! Journal* will inspire you to focus on and achieve your weight loss goals. A few rules of the road:

1: FORGET SPELLING AND PUNCTUATION.
2: WRITE QUICKLY TO WARD OFF YOUR INNER CRITIC.
3: SPEAK FROM YOUR HEART.

Among other things, you can record your hunger at the start of each meal; and your thoughts, observations, and challenges.

For example, you feel energized, your clothes are getting looser, your skin is suddenly glowing. Or you could barely make it through for four hours. The idea is to give you a glimpse of how certain foods make you feel, and what food combinations seem to work best for you.

Recognizing the emotional connection you have with food is critical to losing weight and keeping it off, and this journal is a place for you to explore your relationship to food and pinpoint the psychological hot buttons that will help propel you to a flatter belly. So for each day of the first 28 days of the plan, we've given you an exercise in reflection to help you focus your entry. These Core Confidences are essential to forging a true and fruitful mind–belly connection. Confidence, self-awareness, determination, love, acceptance, compassion, organization—if you have any of these qualities, the Core Confidences will help you tap into and exploit them for your belly's benefit.

Make no mistake: Some of the Core Confidences may not be so fun. Some may ask you to confront difficult personal issues or behaviors you might not be proud of. The Core Confidences will help you uncover your demons, confront them, and fight them.

As you fill out these pages, remember to periodically look back and read what you've written in previous entries. That's how you'll spot behavior patterns and notice your progress. Each Core Confidence builds upon the last, moving you closer and closer to a deeper sense of self-awareness.

If you've read the original *Flat Belly Diet!* book and done the diet, you'll notice that the Core Confidences we've included here repeat those from the original 28-day plan. We did this deliberately so you will be able to see how much you've learned and grown since experiencing the benefits of the Flat Belly way of eating. (And, of course, if you haven't read the original book, we wanted to be sure you had the opportunity to work through all the Core Confidences.)

Once you've finished the 28-day plan, we hope you love the program so much that you'll want to continue. You'll see that we've included the 4-Day Anti-Bloat Jumpstart again on the following pages in case you want to repeat it, but it's optional. You can simply skip over those sections and continue to journal as usual if you prefer.

If you do decide to continue, you'll also find room to create your own Mind Tricks and Core Confidences—or simply repeat the ones you found the most helpful. But, of course, you can write anything in these pages that you find helpful—you can paste in your favorite Flat Belly recipes, keep track of pounds and inches you've lost, or insert photos of yourself looking your best to keep you motivated.

We've included three months' worth of pages in this journal—but we hope you keep eating the *Flat Belly Diet* way for as long as you need to stay slim and healthy for life!

Flat Belly Diet!

> The Four-Day Anti-Bloat Jumpstart

A full 96 hours is all it takes to spark your commitment to the *Flat Belly Diet*—and lose a few pounds! The Jumpstart consists of:

A DAILY DOSE OF SASSY WATER Created by Cynthia, this make-ahead concoction helps guard against dehydration.

A MIND TRICK AT EVERY MEAL Fast mental fixes help get your brain in the *Flat Belly* game.

> The Four-Week Plan

Twenty-eight days of delicious MUFA-packed meals and recipes that you can mix and match. The plan consists of:

FOUR 400-CALORIE MEALS A DAY Choose from our meal selections or recipes, and be sure to make one meal a Snack Pack.

A MUFA AT EVERY MEAL These superhealthy fats keep you feeling full and ensure every meal is exceptionally tasty.

ONE DAILY CORE CONFIDENCE REFLECTION Spend 15 minutes a day exploring your relationship to food and desire to reach your goals.

> An Optional Exercise Program

Fat-burning walks, a Metabolism Boost, and a Belly Routine will help you build muscle and maximize calorie burn.

DAY 1

BREAKFAST

WHAT I ATE:

MUFA: CALORIES:

TIME: HUNGER BEFORE: -5 -3 0 3 5 7 | HUNGER AFTER: -5 -3 0 3 5 7

LUNCH

WHAT I ATE:

MUFA: CALORIES:

TIME: HUNGER BEFORE: -5 -3 0 3 5 7 | HUNGER AFTER: -5 -3 0 3 5 7

SNACK

WHAT I ATE:

MUFA: CALORIES:

TIME: HUNGER BEFORE: -5 -3 0 3 5 7 | HUNGER AFTER: -5 -3 0 3 5 7

DINNER

WHAT I ATE:

MUFA: CALORIES:

TIME: HUNGER BEFORE: -5 -3 0 3 5 7 | HUNGER AFTER: -5 -3 0 3 5 7

CORE CONFIDENCE: Write down at least three reasons why you have chosen to go on the *Flat Belly Diet*. Describe how you feel about the 28 days ahead and what you expect from yourself.

WORKOUT		
WALKING	Fat Blast Walk _____minutes	Calorie Torch Walk _____minutes
STRENGTH TRAINING	The Belly Routine ____sets____reps	The Metabolism Boost ___sets___reps
HOW I FELT:		

DAY 2

BREAKFAST

WHAT I ATE:

MUFA: CALORIES:

TIME: HUNGER BEFORE: -5 -3 0 3 5 7   HUNGER AFTER: -5 -3 0 3 5 7

LUNCH

WHAT I ATE:

MUFA: CALORIES:

TIME: HUNGER BEFORE: -5 -3 0 3 5 7   HUNGER AFTER: -5 -3 0 3 5 7

SNACK

WHAT I ATE:

MUFA: CALORIES:

TIME: HUNGER BEFORE: -5 -3 0 3 5 7   HUNGER AFTER: -5 -3 0 3 5 7

DINNER

WHAT I ATE:

MUFA: CALORIES:

TIME: HUNGER BEFORE: -5 -3 0 3 5 7   HUNGER AFTER: -5 -3 0 3 5 7

CORE CONFIDENCE: List four things that will help you succeed on the *Flat Belly Diet* (example: "my family's cooperation"). Now write about what you are going to do to ensure that you get each of the four things you need.

_____

_____

_____

_____

_____

_____

_____

_____

_____

_____

_____

_____

_____

_____

_____

_____

WORKOUT		
WALKING	Fat Blast Walk _____minutes	Calorie Torch Walk _____minutes
STRENGTH TRAINING	The Belly Routine ____sets____reps	The Metabolism Boost ___sets___reps
HOW I FELT:		

DAY 3

BREAKFAST

WHAT I ATE:

MUFA: CALORIES:

TIME: HUNGER BEFORE: -5 -3 0 3 5 7 | HUNGER AFTER: -5 -3 0 3 5 7

LUNCH

WHAT I ATE:

MUFA: CALORIES:

TIME: HUNGER BEFORE: -5 -3 0 3 5 7 | HUNGER AFTER: -5 -3 0 3 5 7

SNACK

WHAT I ATE:

MUFA: CALORIES:

TIME: HUNGER BEFORE: -5 -3 0 3 5 7 | HUNGER AFTER: -5 -3 0 3 5 7

DINNER

WHAT I ATE:

MUFA: CALORIES:

TIME: HUNGER BEFORE: -5 -3 0 3 5 7 | HUNGER AFTER: -5 -3 0 3 5 7

CORE CONFIDENCE: Practice mindful eating. If you watch TV, check your e-mail, even read the newspaper during meals, you will be distracted from how much and how fast you're eating. Have one meal today in total peace and quiet. Take your time; savor the taste and texture of the food and, eventually, the sensation of fullness. Be conscious of the emotions you feel while you eat. Write about the experience.

_____

_____

_____

_____

_____

_____

_____

_____

_____

_____

_____

_____

_____

_____

_____

_____

_____

WORKOUT		
WALKING	Fat Blast Walk _____minutes	Calorie Torch Walk _____minutes
STRENGTH TRAINING	The Belly Routine ____sets____reps	The Metabolism Boost ___sets___reps

HOW I FELT:

DAY 4

BREAKFAST

WHAT I ATE:

MUFA: CALORIES:

TIME: HUNGER BEFORE: -5 -3 0 3 5 7   HUNGER AFTER: -5 -3 0 3 5 7

LUNCH

WHAT I ATE:

MUFA: CALORIES:

TIME: HUNGER BEFORE: -5 -3 0 3 5 7   HUNGER AFTER: -5 -3 0 3 5 7

SNACK

WHAT I ATE:

MUFA: CALORIES:

TIME: HUNGER BEFORE: -5 -3 0 3 5 7   HUNGER AFTER: -5 -3 0 3 5 7

DINNER

WHAT I ATE:

MUFA: CALORIES:

TIME: HUNGER BEFORE: -5 -3 0 3 5 7   HUNGER AFTER: -5 -3 0 3 5 7

CORE CONFIDENCE: Think of a meal that didn't go well—maybe you overindulged or ate something you later wished you hadn't. Imagine you could go back and "do over" that meal. Write about what you would do differently next time around.

_____

_____

_____

_____

_____

_____

_____

_____

_____

_____

_____

_____

_____

_____

_____

_____

WORKOUT		
WALKING	Fat Blast Walk _____minutes	Calorie Torch Walk _____minutes
STRENGTH TRAINING	The Belly Routine ____sets____reps	The Metabolism Boost ___sets___reps
HOW I FELT:		

DAY 5

BREAKFAST

WHAT I ATE:

MUFA: CALORIES:

TIME: HUNGER BEFORE: -5 -3 0 3 5 7   HUNGER AFTER: -5 -3 0 3 5 7

LUNCH

WHAT I ATE:

MUFA: CALORIES:

TIME: HUNGER BEFORE: -5 -3 0 3 5 7   HUNGER AFTER: -5 -3 0 3 5 7

SNACK

WHAT I ATE:

MUFA: CALORIES:

TIME: HUNGER BEFORE: -5 -3 0 3 5 7   HUNGER AFTER: -5 -3 0 3 5 7

DINNER

WHAT I ATE:

MUFA: CALORIES:

TIME: HUNGER BEFORE: -5 -3 0 3 5 7   HUNGER AFTER: -5 -3 0 3 5 7

■ **CORE CONFIDENCE:** Write down two changes you made during the Four-Day Anti-Bloat Jumpstart. How many of these changes turned out to be easier to make than you expected? Describe what happened in each instance.

_____

_____

_____

_____

_____

_____

_____

_____

_____

_____

_____

_____

_____

_____

_____

_____

WORKOUT		
WALKING	Fat Blast Walk _____minutes	Calorie Torch Walk _____minutes
STRENGTH TRAINING	The Belly Routine ____sets____reps	The Metabolism Boost ___sets___reps

HOW I FELT:

DAY 6

BREAKFAST

WHAT I ATE:

MUFA: CALORIES:

TIME: HUNGER BEFORE: -5 -3 0 3 5 7 | HUNGER AFTER: -5 -3 0 3 5 7

LUNCH

WHAT I ATE:

MUFA: CALORIES:

TIME: HUNGER BEFORE: -5 -3 0 3 5 7 | HUNGER AFTER: -5 -3 0 3 5 7

SNACK

WHAT I ATE:

MUFA: CALORIES:

TIME: HUNGER BEFORE: -5 -3 0 3 5 7 | HUNGER AFTER: -5 -3 0 3 5 7

DINNER

WHAT I ATE:

MUFA: CALORIES:

TIME: HUNGER BEFORE: -5 -3 0 3 5 7 | HUNGER AFTER: -5 -3 0 3 5 7

CORE CONFIDENCE: Today, see if you can tell the difference between how it feels to eat when you're feeling hungry and how it feels to eat when you're feeling stressed. Write about those reflections.

_____

_____

_____

_____

_____

_____

_____

_____

_____

_____

_____

_____

_____

_____

_____

_____

WORKOUT		
WALKING	Fat Blast Walk _____minutes	Calorie Torch Walk _____minutes
STRENGTH TRAINING	The Belly Routine ____sets____reps	The Metabolism Boost ___sets___reps
HOW I FELT:		

DAY 7

BREAKFAST

WHAT I ATE:

MUFA: CALORIES:

TIME: HUNGER BEFORE: -5 -3 0 3 5 7   HUNGER AFTER: -5 -3 0 3 5 7

LUNCH

WHAT I ATE:

MUFA: CALORIES:

TIME: HUNGER BEFORE: -5 -3 0 3 5 7   HUNGER AFTER: -5 -3 0 3 5 7

SNACK

WHAT I ATE:

MUFA: CALORIES:

TIME: HUNGER BEFORE: -5 -3 0 3 5 7   HUNGER AFTER: -5 -3 0 3 5 7

DINNER

WHAT I ATE:

MUFA: CALORIES:

TIME: HUNGER BEFORE: -5 -3 0 3 5 7   HUNGER AFTER: -5 -3 0 3 5 7

CORE CONFIDENCE: Today you cross the finish line for Week One. Well done! List the two or three things you found most difficult about being on the *Flat Belly Diet*. Now write about what you're going to do to clear those hurdles in the week ahead.

_____

_____

_____

_____

_____

_____

_____

_____

_____

_____

_____

_____

_____

_____

_____

_____

_____

_____

WORKOUT		
WALKING	Fat Blast Walk _____minutes	Calorie Torch Walk _____minutes
STRENGTH TRAINING	The Belly Routine ____sets____reps	The Metabolism Boost ___sets___reps
HOW I FELT:		

DAY 8

BREAKFAST

WHAT I ATE:

MUFA: CALORIES:

TIME: HUNGER BEFORE: -5 -3 0 3 5 7   HUNGER AFTER: -5 -3 0 3 5 7

LUNCH

WHAT I ATE:

MUFA: CALORIES:

TIME: HUNGER BEFORE: -5 -3 0 3 5 7   HUNGER AFTER: -5 -3 0 3 5 7

SNACK

WHAT I ATE:

MUFA: CALORIES:

TIME: HUNGER BEFORE: -5 -3 0 3 5 7   HUNGER AFTER: -5 -3 0 3 5 7

DINNER

WHAT I ATE:

MUFA: CALORIES:

TIME: HUNGER BEFORE: -5 -3 0 3 5 7   HUNGER AFTER: -5 -3 0 3 5 7

CORE CONFIDENCE: Write a personal bio. Who are you? What personal strengths do you bring to your job, family, and health? Then write a bio on the person you aspire to be. Is she more confident, more active, more compassionate? What qualities can you take from the first to help you become the second?

WORKOUT	
WALKING	Fat Blast Walk _____minutes	Calorie Torch Walk _____minutes
STRENGTH TRAINING	The Belly Routine ____sets____reps	The Metabolism Boost ___sets___reps

HOW I FELT:

DAY 9

BREAKFAST

WHAT I ATE:

MUFA: CALORIES:

TIME: HUNGER BEFORE: -5 -3 0 3 5 7   HUNGER AFTER: -5 -3 0 3 5 7

LUNCH

WHAT I ATE:

MUFA: CALORIES:

TIME: HUNGER BEFORE: -5 -3 0 3 5 7   HUNGER AFTER: -5 -3 0 3 5 7

SNACK

WHAT I ATE:

MUFA: CALORIES:

TIME: HUNGER BEFORE: -5 -3 0 3 5 7   HUNGER AFTER: -5 -3 0 3 5 7

DINNER

WHAT I ATE:

MUFA: CALORIES:

TIME: HUNGER BEFORE: -5 -3 0 3 5 7   HUNGER AFTER: -5 -3 0 3 5 7

CORE CONFIDENCE: Think back over the last few days. Identify one food-related faux pas (maybe you snuck a few Hershey's kisses from the receptionist's desk at work), and write that on the left side of the page. On the opposite side of the page, jot down everything you can think of that you did right that day (made your child laugh, started a project, took a long walk). Now take another look at the "big picture" of your day. Do you see the one setback in a different light?

WORKOUT		
WALKING	Fat Blast Walk _____ minutes	Calorie Torch Walk _____ minutes
STRENGTH TRAINING	The Belly Routine ____ sets ____ reps	The Metabolism Boost ___ sets ___ reps
HOW I FELT:		

DAY 10

BREAKFAST

WHAT I ATE:

MUFA: CALORIES:

TIME: HUNGER BEFORE: -5 -3 0 3 5 7   HUNGER AFTER: -5 -3 0 3 5 7

LUNCH

WHAT I ATE:

MUFA: CALORIES:

TIME: HUNGER BEFORE: -5 -3 0 3 5 7   HUNGER AFTER: -5 -3 0 3 5 7

SNACK

WHAT I ATE:

MUFA: CALORIES:

TIME: HUNGER BEFORE: -5 -3 0 3 5 7   HUNGER AFTER: -5 -3 0 3 5 7

DINNER

WHAT I ATE:

MUFA: CALORIES:

TIME: HUNGER BEFORE: -5 -3 0 3 5 7   HUNGER AFTER: -5 -3 0 3 5 7

CORE CONFIDENCE: Today let's focus on what you're grateful for. Keep listing what you love about your body, your family, your job—even your personal surroundings—until your space is filled.

_____

_____

_____

_____

_____

_____

_____

_____

_____

_____

_____

_____

_____

_____

_____

_____

WORKOUT	
WALKING	Fat Blast Walk _____minutes	Calorie Torch Walk _____minutes
STRENGTH TRAINING	The Belly Routine ____sets____reps	The Metabolism Boost ___sets___reps
HOW I FELT:		

DAY 11

BREAKFAST

WHAT I ATE:

MUFA: CALORIES:

TIME: | HUNGER BEFORE: -5 -3 0 3 5 7 | HUNGER AFTER: -5 -3 0 3 5 7

LUNCH

WHAT I ATE:

MUFA: CALORIES:

TIME: | HUNGER BEFORE: -5 -3 0 3 5 7 | HUNGER AFTER: -5 -3 0 3 5 7

SNACK

WHAT I ATE:

MUFA: CALORIES:

TIME: | HUNGER BEFORE: -5 -3 0 3 5 7 | HUNGER AFTER: -5 -3 0 3 5 7

DINNER

WHAT I ATE:

MUFA: CALORIES:

TIME: | HUNGER BEFORE: -5 -3 0 3 5 7 | HUNGER AFTER: -5 -3 0 3 5 7

CORE CONFIDENCE: Create a list of five instant indulgences that can be substituted for food when cravings or emotions threaten to get the best of you.

_____

_____

_____

_____

_____

_____

_____

_____

_____

_____

_____

_____

_____

_____

_____

_____

WORKOUT	
WALKING	Fat Blast Walk _____minutes	Calorie Torch Walk _____minutes
STRENGTH TRAINING	The Belly Routine ____sets____reps	The Metabolism Boost ___sets___reps

HOW I FELT:

DAY 12

BREAKFAST

WHAT I ATE:

MUFA: CALORIES:

TIME: HUNGER BEFORE: -5 -3 0 3 5 7   HUNGER AFTER: -5 -3 0 3 5 7

LUNCH

WHAT I ATE:

MUFA: CALORIES:

TIME: HUNGER BEFORE: -5 -3 0 3 5 7   HUNGER AFTER: -5 -3 0 3 5 7

SNACK

WHAT I ATE:

MUFA: CALORIES:

TIME: HUNGER BEFORE: -5 -3 0 3 5 7   HUNGER AFTER: -5 -3 0 3 5 7

DINNER

WHAT I ATE:

MUFA: CALORIES:

TIME: HUNGER BEFORE: -5 -3 0 3 5 7   HUNGER AFTER: -5 -3 0 3 5 7

CORE CONFIDENCE: Write a love note to your belly. Include at least two reasons it deserves your affection and respect.

_____

_____

_____

_____

_____

_____

_____

_____

_____

_____

_____

_____

_____

_____

_____

_____

WORKOUT	
WALKING	Fat Blast Walk _____minutes	Calorie Torch Walk _____minutes
STRENGTH TRAINING	The Belly Routine ____sets____reps	The Metabolism Boost ___sets___reps

HOW I FELT:

DAY 13

BREAKFAST

WHAT I ATE:

MUFA: CALORIES:

TIME: | HUNGER BEFORE: -5 -3 0 3 5 7 | HUNGER AFTER: -5 -3 0 3 5 7

LUNCH

WHAT I ATE:

MUFA: CALORIES:

TIME: | HUNGER BEFORE: -5 -3 0 3 5 7 | HUNGER AFTER: -5 -3 0 3 5 7

SNACK

WHAT I ATE:

MUFA: CALORIES:

TIME: | HUNGER BEFORE: -5 -3 0 3 5 7 | HUNGER AFTER: -5 -3 0 3 5 7

DINNER

WHAT I ATE:

MUFA: CALORIES:

TIME: | HUNGER BEFORE: -5 -3 0 3 5 7 | HUNGER AFTER: -5 -3 0 3 5 7

▧ **CORE CONFIDENCE:** To learn more about your food/feelings connection, make four columns, labeled **anger, sadness, fear,** and **happiness**. Remember the last couple of times you craved a food when you were experiencing each of those emotions. Think about what you craved—and ate—and note it in the appropriate column.

WORKOUT	
WALKING	Fat Blast Walk _____minutes	Calorie Torch Walk _____minutes
STRENGTH TRAINING	The Belly Routine ____sets____reps	The Metabolism Boost ___sets___reps

HOW I FELT:

DAY 14

BREAKFAST

WHAT I ATE:

MUFA: CALORIES:

TIME: HUNGER BEFORE: -5 -3 0 3 5 7   HUNGER AFTER: -5 -3 0 3 5 7

LUNCH

WHAT I ATE:

MUFA: CALORIES:

TIME: HUNGER BEFORE: -5 -3 0 3 5 7   HUNGER AFTER: -5 -3 0 3 5 7

SNACK

WHAT I ATE:

MUFA: CALORIES:

TIME: HUNGER BEFORE: -5 -3 0 3 5 7   HUNGER AFTER: -5 -3 0 3 5 7

DINNER

WHAT I ATE:

MUFA: CALORIES:

TIME: HUNGER BEFORE: -5 -3 0 3 5 7   HUNGER AFTER: -5 -3 0 3 5 7

CORE CONFIDENCE: You've just finished Week Two! Congratulations—you're halfway there! Write about how you feel reaching this milestone. Describe the changes you have noticed this week in yourself and your attitudes toward food and your body—your belly in particular. Outline your expectations for the week ahead.

_____

_____

_____

_____

_____

_____

_____

_____

_____

_____

_____

_____

_____

_____

_____

_____

WORKOUT		
WALKING	Fat Blast Walk _____minutes	Calorie Torch Walk _____minutes
STRENGTH TRAINING	The Belly Routine ____sets____reps	The Metabolism Boost ___sets___reps
HOW I FELT:		

DAY 15

BREAKFAST

WHAT I ATE:

MUFA: CALORIES:

TIME: HUNGER BEFORE: -5 -3 0 3 5 7   HUNGER AFTER: -5 -3 0 3 5 7

LUNCH

WHAT I ATE:

MUFA: CALORIES:

TIME: HUNGER BEFORE: -5 -3 0 3 5 7   HUNGER AFTER: -5 -3 0 3 5 7

SNACK

WHAT I ATE:

MUFA: CALORIES:

TIME: HUNGER BEFORE: -5 -3 0 3 5 7   HUNGER AFTER: -5 -3 0 3 5 7

DINNER

WHAT I ATE:

MUFA: CALORIES:

TIME: HUNGER BEFORE: -5 -3 0 3 5 7   HUNGER AFTER: -5 -3 0 3 5 7

CORE CONFIDENCE: Identify three or four "high-risk" scenarios— occasions, activities, or places in which you are in danger of eating more than you should or eating the wrong foods. Now create an escape plan that you can implement to avert trouble in each scenario. Write up a description of this plan, using an "If X, then I'll Y" format.

_____

_____

_____

_____

_____

_____

_____

_____

_____

_____

_____

_____

_____

_____

_____

_____

_____

WORKOUT

WALKING	Fat Blast Walk _____minutes	Calorie Torch Walk _____minutes
STRENGTH TRAINING	The Belly Routine ____sets____reps	The Metabolism Boost ___sets___reps

HOW I FELT:

DAY 16

BREAKFAST

WHAT I ATE:

MUFA: CALORIES:

TIME: HUNGER BEFORE: -5 -3 0 3 5 7   HUNGER AFTER: -5 -3 0 3 5 7

LUNCH

WHAT I ATE:

MUFA: CALORIES:

TIME: HUNGER BEFORE: -5 -3 0 3 5 7   HUNGER AFTER: -5 -3 0 3 5 7

SNACK

WHAT I ATE:

MUFA: CALORIES:

TIME: HUNGER BEFORE: -5 -3 0 3 5 7   HUNGER AFTER: -5 -3 0 3 5 7

DINNER

WHAT I ATE:

MUFA: CALORIES:

TIME: HUNGER BEFORE: -5 -3 0 3 5 7   HUNGER AFTER: -5 -3 0 3 5 7

CORE CONFIDENCE: Make a list of at least five activities you've always been interested in but never managed to get around to doing. Rank them in order of preference. Then, alongside each item, enter the very first action you need to take to begin to make it happen.

_____

_____

_____

_____

_____

_____

_____

_____

_____

_____

_____

_____

_____

_____

_____

_____

WORKOUT	
WALKING	Fat Blast Walk _____ minutes	Calorie Torch Walk _____ minutes
STRENGTH TRAINING	The Belly Routine ____ sets ____ reps	The Metabolism Boost ___ sets ___ reps

HOW I FELT:

DAY 17

BREAKFAST

WHAT I ATE:

MUFA: CALORIES:

TIME: HUNGER BEFORE: -5 -3 0 3 5 7   HUNGER AFTER: -5 -3 0 3 5 7

LUNCH

WHAT I ATE:

MUFA: CALORIES:

TIME: HUNGER BEFORE: -5 -3 0 3 5 7   HUNGER AFTER: -5 -3 0 3 5 7

SNACK

WHAT I ATE:

MUFA: CALORIES:

TIME: HUNGER BEFORE: -5 -3 0 3 5 7   HUNGER AFTER: -5 -3 0 3 5 7

DINNER

WHAT I ATE:

MUFA: CALORIES:

TIME: HUNGER BEFORE: -5 -3 0 3 5 7   HUNGER AFTER: -5 -3 0 3 5 7

CORE CONFIDENCE: Plumb your memory banks for unhealthy eating rules you used to follow (like always cleaning your plate). Where did you learn those rules? How do they continue to affect the way you eat? Now write your "New Rules to Eat By" (for example, "Listen to my stomach and stop eating when it's full").

WORKOUT

WALKING	Fat Blast Walk _____minutes	Calorie Torch Walk _____minutes
STRENGTH TRAINING	The Belly Routine ____sets____reps	The Metabolism Boost ___sets___reps

HOW I FELT:

DAY 18

BREAKFAST

WHAT I ATE:

MUFA: CALORIES:

TIME: HUNGER BEFORE: -5 -3 0 3 5 7   HUNGER AFTER: -5 -3 0 3 5 7

LUNCH

WHAT I ATE:

MUFA: CALORIES:

TIME: HUNGER BEFORE: -5 -3 0 3 5 7   HUNGER AFTER: -5 -3 0 3 5 7

SNACK

WHAT I ATE:

MUFA: CALORIES:

TIME: HUNGER BEFORE: -5 -3 0 3 5 7   HUNGER AFTER: -5 -3 0 3 5 7

DINNER

WHAT I ATE:

MUFA: CALORIES:

TIME: HUNGER BEFORE: -5 -3 0 3 5 7   HUNGER AFTER: -5 -3 0 3 5 7

CORE CONFIDENCE: Make a list of all the things and people you're angry with. Then write next to each, in capital letters: I FORGIVE YOU.

_____

_____

_____

_____

_____

_____

_____

_____

_____

_____

_____

_____

_____

_____

_____

_____

WORKOUT

WALKING	Fat Blast Walk _____minutes	Calorie Torch Walk _____minutes
STRENGTH TRAINING	The Belly Routine ____sets____reps	The Metabolism Boost ___sets___reps

HOW I FELT:

DAY 19

BREAKFAST

WHAT I ATE:

MUFA: CALORIES:

TIME: | HUNGER BEFORE: -5 -3 0 3 5 7 | HUNGER AFTER: -5 -3 0 3 5 7

LUNCH

WHAT I ATE:

MUFA: CALORIES:

TIME: | HUNGER BEFORE: -5 -3 0 3 5 7 | HUNGER AFTER: -5 -3 0 3 5 7

SNACK

WHAT I ATE:

MUFA: CALORIES:

TIME: | HUNGER BEFORE: -5 -3 0 3 5 7 | HUNGER AFTER: -5 -3 0 3 5 7

DINNER

WHAT I ATE:

MUFA: CALORIES:

TIME: | HUNGER BEFORE: -5 -3 0 3 5 7 | HUNGER AFTER: -5 -3 0 3 5 7

CORE CONFIDENCE: Try to go through the day appreciating how very much you have. Make a list of five moments you're most grateful for today; read it before you go to sleep.

_____

_____

_____

_____

_____

_____

_____

_____

_____

_____

_____

_____

_____

_____

_____

_____

_____

_____

WORKOUT

WALKING	Fat Blast Walk _____minutes	Calorie Torch Walk _____minutes
STRENGTH TRAINING	The Belly Routine ____sets____reps	The Metabolism Boost ___sets___reps
HOW I FELT:		

DAY 20

BREAKFAST

WHAT I ATE:

MUFA: CALORIES:

TIME: HUNGER BEFORE: -5 -3 0 3 5 7 | HUNGER AFTER: -5 -3 0 3 5 7

LUNCH

WHAT I ATE:

MUFA: CALORIES:

TIME: HUNGER BEFORE: -5 -3 0 3 5 7 | HUNGER AFTER: -5 -3 0 3 5 7

SNACK

WHAT I ATE:

MUFA: CALORIES:

TIME: HUNGER BEFORE: -5 -3 0 3 5 7 | HUNGER AFTER: -5 -3 0 3 5 7

DINNER

WHAT I ATE:

MUFA: CALORIES:

TIME: HUNGER BEFORE: -5 -3 0 3 5 7 | HUNGER AFTER: -5 -3 0 3 5 7

CORE CONFIDENCE: Give yourself a confidence boost. Make a list of all the new things you're doing that you weren't doing 3 weeks ago. You've probably accomplished a lot more than you think.

_____

_____

_____

_____

_____

_____

_____

_____

_____

_____

_____

_____

_____

_____

_____

WORKOUT		
WALKING	Fat Blast Walk _____minutes	Calorie Torch Walk _____minutes
STRENGTH TRAINING	The Belly Routine ____sets____reps	The Metabolism Boost ___sets___reps
HOW I FELT:		

DAY 21

BREAKFAST

WHAT I ATE:

MUFA: CALORIES:

TIME: HUNGER BEFORE: -5 -3 0 3 5 7   HUNGER AFTER: -5 -3 0 3 5 7

LUNCH

WHAT I ATE:

MUFA: CALORIES:

TIME: HUNGER BEFORE: -5 -3 0 3 5 7   HUNGER AFTER: -5 -3 0 3 5 7

SNACK

WHAT I ATE:

MUFA: CALORIES:

TIME: HUNGER BEFORE: -5 -3 0 3 5 7   HUNGER AFTER: -5 -3 0 3 5 7

DINNER

WHAT I ATE:

MUFA: CALORIES:

TIME: HUNGER BEFORE: -5 -3 0 3 5 7   HUNGER AFTER: -5 -3 0 3 5 7

CORE CONFIDENCE: Welcome to the end of Week Three! Write about how it feels to have come so far. Do you feel empowered? Invincible? Proud? Connected to your belly? Write down all the compliments you've received—including thoughts you've had yourself about how far you've come and how great you look.

WORKOUT	
WALKING	Fat Blast Walk _____minutes

WALKING	Fat Blast Walk _____minutes	Calorie Torch Walk _____minutes
STRENGTH TRAINING	The Belly Routine ____sets____reps	The Metabolism Boost ___sets___reps

HOW I FELT:

DAY 22

BREAKFAST

WHAT I ATE:

MUFA: CALORIES:

TIME: HUNGER BEFORE: -5 -3 0 3 5 7   HUNGER AFTER: -5 -3 0 3 5 7

LUNCH

WHAT I ATE:

MUFA: CALORIES:

TIME: HUNGER BEFORE: -5 -3 0 3 5 7   HUNGER AFTER: -5 -3 0 3 5 7

SNACK

WHAT I ATE:

MUFA: CALORIES:

TIME: HUNGER BEFORE: -5 -3 0 3 5 7   HUNGER AFTER: -5 -3 0 3 5 7

DINNER

WHAT I ATE:

MUFA: CALORIES:

TIME: HUNGER BEFORE: -5 -3 0 3 5 7   HUNGER AFTER: -5 -3 0 3 5 7

CORE CONFIDENCE: Write today's entry sitting in front of a mirror. Describe who you see as if you were explaining to a friend what this woman looks like. Be as complimentary as possible.

_____

_____

_____

_____

_____

_____

_____

_____

_____

_____

_____

_____

_____

_____

_____

WORKOUT		
WALKING	Fat Blast Walk _____minutes	Calorie Torch Walk _____minutes
STRENGTH TRAINING	The Belly Routine ____sets____reps	The Metabolism Boost ___sets___reps

HOW I FELT:

DAY 23

BREAKFAST

WHAT I ATE:

MUFA: CALORIES:

TIME: HUNGER BEFORE: -5 -3 0 3 5 7 | HUNGER AFTER: -5 -3 0 3 5 7

LUNCH

WHAT I ATE:

MUFA: CALORIES:

TIME: HUNGER BEFORE: -5 -3 0 3 5 7 | HUNGER AFTER: -5 -3 0 3 5 7

SNACK

WHAT I ATE:

MUFA: CALORIES:

TIME: HUNGER BEFORE: -5 -3 0 3 5 7 | HUNGER AFTER: -5 -3 0 3 5 7

DINNER

WHAT I ATE:

MUFA: CALORIES:

TIME: HUNGER BEFORE: -5 -3 0 3 5 7 | HUNGER AFTER: -5 -3 0 3 5 7

CORE CONFIDENCE: If you could have only three foods for the rest of your life, what would they be? Think of a quick recipe—how can you make them fit into the *Flat Belly Diet*?

_____

_____

_____

_____

_____

_____

_____

_____

_____

_____

_____

_____

_____

_____

_____

_____

_____

_____

WORKOUT	
WALKING	Fat Blast Walk _____minutes	Calorie Torch Walk _____minutes
STRENGTH TRAINING	The Belly Routine ____sets____reps	The Metabolism Boost ___sets___reps

HOW I FELT:

DAY 24

BREAKFAST

WHAT I ATE:

MUFA: CALORIES:

TIME: | HUNGER BEFORE: -5 -3 0 3 5 7 | HUNGER AFTER: -5 -3 0 3 5 7

LUNCH

WHAT I ATE:

MUFA: CALORIES:

TIME: | HUNGER BEFORE: -5 -3 0 3 5 7 | HUNGER AFTER: -5 -3 0 3 5 7

SNACK

WHAT I ATE:

MUFA: CALORIES:

TIME: | HUNGER BEFORE: -5 -3 0 3 5 7 | HUNGER AFTER: -5 -3 0 3 5 7

DINNER

WHAT I ATE:

MUFA: CALORIES:

TIME: | HUNGER BEFORE: -5 -3 0 3 5 7 | HUNGER AFTER: -5 -3 0 3 5 7

CORE CONFIDENCE: In three columns labeled **high, medium,** and **low**, list your motivators in the appropriate column. For example, going down a dress size and being able to walk up a flight of stairs without feeling winded may rank high, while getting a better night's sleep might be a medium.

WORKOUT		
WALKING	Fat Blast Walk _____minutes	Calorie Torch Walk _____minutes
STRENGTH TRAINING	The Belly Routine ____sets____reps	The Metabolism Boost ___sets___reps
HOW I FELT:		

DAY 25

BREAKFAST

WHAT I ATE:

MUFA: CALORIES:

TIME: HUNGER BEFORE: -5 -3 0 3 5 7   HUNGER AFTER: -5 -3 0 3 5 7

LUNCH

WHAT I ATE:

MUFA: CALORIES:

TIME: HUNGER BEFORE: -5 -3 0 3 5 7   HUNGER AFTER: -5 -3 0 3 5 7

SNACK

WHAT I ATE:

MUFA: CALORIES:

TIME: HUNGER BEFORE: -5 -3 0 3 5 7   HUNGER AFTER: -5 -3 0 3 5 7

DINNER

WHAT I ATE:

MUFA: CALORIES:

TIME: HUNGER BEFORE: -5 -3 0 3 5 7   HUNGER AFTER: -5 -3 0 3 5 7

CORE CONFIDENCE: Describe a failure in your recent past. How did you get through it? What was the number one thing that helped you persevere? How can you apply this to your experience on the *Flat Belly Diet*?

_____

_____

_____

_____

_____

_____

_____

_____

_____

_____

_____

_____

_____

_____

_____

_____

WORKOUT		
WALKING	Fat Blast Walk _____minutes	Calorie Torch Walk _____minutes
STRENGTH TRAINING	The Belly Routine ____sets____reps	The Metabolism Boost ___sets___reps

HOW I FELT:

DAY 26

BREAKFAST

WHAT I ATE:

MUFA: CALORIES:

TIME: HUNGER BEFORE: -5 -3 0 3 5 7   HUNGER AFTER: -5 -3 0 3 5 7

LUNCH

WHAT I ATE:

MUFA: CALORIES:

TIME: HUNGER BEFORE: -5 -3 0 3 5 7   HUNGER AFTER: -5 -3 0 3 5 7

SNACK

WHAT I ATE:

MUFA: CALORIES:

TIME: HUNGER BEFORE: -5 -3 0 3 5 7   HUNGER AFTER: -5 -3 0 3 5 7

DINNER

WHAT I ATE:

MUFA: CALORIES:

TIME: HUNGER BEFORE: -5 -3 0 3 5 7   HUNGER AFTER: -5 -3 0 3 5 7

CORE CONFIDENCE: Write about a woman you admire. Why is she so special to you? If you could absorb two of her qualities, what would they be and why?

_____

_____

_____

_____

_____

_____

_____

_____

_____

_____

_____

_____

_____

_____

_____

_____

WORKOUT		
WALKING	Fat Blast Walk _____minutes	Calorie Torch Walk _____minutes
STRENGTH TRAINING	The Belly Routine ____sets____reps	The Metabolism Boost ___sets___reps

HOW I FELT:

DAY 27

BREAKFAST

WHAT I ATE:

MUFA: CALORIES:

TIME: HUNGER BEFORE: -5 -3 0 3 5 7   HUNGER AFTER: -5 -3 0 3 5 7

LUNCH

WHAT I ATE:

MUFA: CALORIES:

TIME: HUNGER BEFORE: -5 -3 0 3 5 7   HUNGER AFTER: -5 -3 0 3 5 7

SNACK

WHAT I ATE:

MUFA: CALORIES:

TIME: HUNGER BEFORE: -5 -3 0 3 5 7   HUNGER AFTER: -5 -3 0 3 5 7

DINNER

WHAT I ATE:

MUFA: CALORIES:

TIME: HUNGER BEFORE: -5 -3 0 3 5 7   HUNGER AFTER: -5 -3 0 3 5 7

▒ **CORE CONFIDENCE:** Create a diet motivation booster list: Write down all of the reasons you chose the *Flat Belly Diet*. Be sure to include what you'll get out of changing that's important to you, both **today** and in the **future**. For example: **today**—feel lighter and more energized; **future**—not have to take medication. Reread it periodically as a reminder of something you did for yourself.

_____

_____

_____

_____

_____

_____

_____

_____

_____

_____

_____

_____

_____

_____

_____

_____

_____

WORKOUT

WALKING	Fat Blast Walk _____minutes	Calorie Torch Walk _____minutes
STRENGTH TRAINING	The Belly Routine ____sets____reps	The Metabolism Boost ___sets___reps
HOW I FELT:		

DAY 28

BREAKFAST

WHAT I ATE:

MUFA: CALORIES:

TIME: HUNGER BEFORE: -5 -3 0 3 5 7   HUNGER AFTER: -5 -3 0 3 5 7

LUNCH

WHAT I ATE:

MUFA: CALORIES:

TIME: HUNGER BEFORE: -5 -3 0 3 5 7   HUNGER AFTER: -5 -3 0 3 5 7

SNACK

WHAT I ATE:

MUFA: CALORIES:

TIME: HUNGER BEFORE: -5 -3 0 3 5 7   HUNGER AFTER: -5 -3 0 3 5 7

DINNER

WHAT I ATE:

MUFA: CALORIES:

TIME: HUNGER BEFORE: -5 -3 0 3 5 7   HUNGER AFTER: -5 -3 0 3 5 7

CORE CONFIDENCE: Congratulations!!! You've reached the end of the formal Four-Week Plan. Describe how it feels to have set out to complete this program and to actually reach your goal. How healthy do you feel? How happy are you with your results? Write a pledge to yourself that you will continue to fuel your body and your mind in this healthy way.

_____

_____

_____

_____

_____

_____

_____

_____

_____

_____

_____

_____

_____

_____

_____

_____

WORKOUT		
WALKING	Fat Blast Walk _____minutes	Calorie Torch Walk _____minutes
STRENGTH TRAINING	The Belly Routine ____sets____reps	The Metabolism Boost ___sets___reps

HOW I FELT:

THE FOUR-DAY ANTI-BLOAT MENU, DAY 1

DATE:

BREAKFAST

- ❏ 1 cup unsweetened cornflakes
- ❏ 1 cup skim milk
- ❏ ½ cup unsweetened applesauce
- ❏ ¼ cup roasted or raw unsalted sunflower seeds
- ❏ Glass of Sassy Water

MIND TRICK:

LUNCH

- ❏ 4 oz organic deli turkey, rolled up
- ❏ 1 low-fat string cheese
- ❏ 1 pint fresh grape tomatoes
- ❏ Glass of Sassy Water

MIND TRICK:

SNACK

- ❏ Blueberry Smoothie: Blend 1 cup skim milk and 1 cup frozen unsweetened blueberries in blender for 1 minute. Transfer to glass and stir in 1 Tbsp cold-pressed organic flaxseed oil, or serve with 1 Tbsp sunflower or pumpkin seeds.

MIND TRICK:

DINNER

- ❏ 1 cup cooked green beans
- ❏ 4 oz grilled tilapia
- ❏ ½ cup roasted red potatoes drizzled with 1 tsp olive oil
- ❏ Glass of Sassy Water

MIND TRICK:

JOURNAL, DAY 1

DATE:

BREAKFAST	
MOOD:	THOUGHTS/CHALLENGES:
HUNGER BEFORE: -5 -3 0 3 5 7	HUNGER AFTER: -5 -3 0 3 5 7

LUNCH	
MOOD:	THOUGHTS/CHALLENGES:
HUNGER BEFORE: -5 -3 0 3 5 7	HUNGER AFTER: -5 -3 0 3 5 7

SNACK	
MOOD:	THOUGHTS/CHALLENGES:
HUNGER BEFORE: -5 -3 0 3 5 7	HUNGER AFTER: -5 -3 0 3 5 7

DINNER	
MOOD:	THOUGHTS/CHALLENGES:
HUNGER BEFORE: -5 -3 0 3 5 7	HUNGER AFTER: -5 -3 0 3 5 7

Hunger Rating

–5 = STARVING. You want to devour the first thing you see and have a hard time slowing down.

–3 = OVERLY HUNGRY AND IRRITABLE. You feel like you waited too long to eat.

0 = MILD TO MODERATE HUNGER. You may have physical symptoms of hunger, like a growling tummy and that "I need to eat soon" feeling, but you aren't starving or experiencing any unpleasant symptoms such as a headache or shaking.

3 = HUNGER BUT NOT CRAVING FREE. You're full, but you don't feel quite satisfied; your thoughts are still focused on food.

5 = JUST RIGHT. Your hunger is gone, and you feel satisfied. Your mind is off food, and you're ready to take on the next task. You feel energized.

7 = A LITTLE TOO MUCH. You think you overdid it. Your tummy feels stretched and uncomfortable. You feel kind of sluggish.

THE FOUR-DAY ANTI-BLOAT MENU, DAY 2

DATE:

BREAKFAST	
❑ 1 cup unsweetened puffed rice cereal	**MIND TRICK:**
❑ 1 cup skim milk	
❑ ¼ cup roasted or raw unsalted sunflower seeds	
❑ 4 oz pineapple tidbits canned in juice	
❑ Glass of Sassy Water	

LUNCH	
❑ 3 oz chunk light tuna in water	**MIND TRICK:**
❑ 1 cup steamed baby carrots	
❑ 1 low-fat string cheese	
❑ Glass of Sassy Water	

SNACK	
❑ Pineapple Smoothie: Blend 1 cup skim milk, 4 oz canned pineapple tidbits in juice, and a handful of ice in blender for 1 minute. Transfer to glass and stir in 1 Tbsp cold-pressed organic flaxseed oil, or serve with 1 Tbsp sunflower or pumpkin seeds.	**MIND TRICK:**

DINNER	
❑ 1 cup fresh cremini mushrooms sautéed with 1 tsp olive oil	**MIND TRICK:**
❑ 3 oz grilled chicken breast	
❑ ½ cup cooked brown rice	
❑ Glass of Sassy Water	

JOURNAL, DAY 2

DATE:

BREAKFAST	
MOOD:	THOUGHTS/CHALLENGES:

HUNGER BEFORE:
-5 -3 0 3 5 7

HUNGER AFTER:
-5 -3 0 3 5 7

LUNCH	
MOOD:	THOUGHTS/CHALLENGES:

HUNGER BEFORE:
-5 -3 0 3 5 7

HUNGER AFTER:
-5 -3 0 3 5 7

SNACK	
MOOD:	THOUGHTS/CHALLENGES:

HUNGER BEFORE:
-5 -3 0 3 5 7

HUNGER AFTER:
-5 -3 0 3 5 7

DINNER	
MOOD:	THOUGHTS/CHALLENGES:

HUNGER BEFORE:
-5 -3 0 3 5 7

HUNGER AFTER:
-5 -3 0 3 5 7

Hunger Rating

–5 = STARVING. You want to devour the first thing you see and have a hard time slowing down.

–3 = OVERLY HUNGRY AND IRRITABLE. You feel like you waited too long to eat.

0 = MILD TO MODERATE HUNGER. You may have physical symptoms of hunger, like a growling tummy and that "I need to eat soon" feeling, but you aren't starving or experiencing any unpleasant symptoms such as a headache or shaking.

3 = HUNGER BUT NOT CRAVING FREE. You're full, but you don't feel quite satisfied; your thoughts are still focused on food.

5 = JUST RIGHT. Your hunger is gone, and you feel satisfied. Your mind is off food, and you're ready to take on the next task. You feel energized.

7 = A LITTLE TOO MUCH. You think you overdid it. Your tummy feels stretched and uncomfortable. You feel kind of sluggish.

THE FOUR-DAY ANTI-BLOAT MENU, DAY 3

DATE:

BREAKFAST	
❑ 1 cup unsweetened cornflakes	**MIND TRICK:**
❑ 1 cup skim milk	
❑ ¼ cup roasted or raw unsalted sunflower seeds	
❑ 2 Tbsp raisins	
❑ Glass of Sassy Water	

LUNCH	
❑ 4 oz organic deli turkey, rolled up	**MIND TRICK:**
❑ 1 low-fat string cheese	
❑ 1 pint grape tomatoes	
❑ Glass of Sassy Water	

SNACK	
❑ Peach Smoothie: Blend 1 cup skim milk and 1 cup frozen unsweetened peaches in blender for 1 minute. Transfer to glass and stir in 1 Tbsp cold-pressed organic flaxseed oil, or serve with 1 Tbsp sunflower or pumpkin seeds.	**MIND TRICK:**

DINNER	
❑ 1 cup cooked green beans	**MIND TRICK:**
❑ 3 oz grilled or baked turkey breast cutlet	
❑ ½ cup roasted red potatoes drizzled with 1 tsp olive oil	
❑ Glass of Sassy Water	

JOURNAL, DAY 3

DATE:

BREAKFAST	
MOOD:	THOUGHTS/CHALLENGES:

HUNGER BEFORE:
-5 -3 0 3 5 7

HUNGER AFTER:
-5 -3 0 3 5 7

LUNCH	
MOOD:	THOUGHTS/CHALLENGES:

HUNGER BEFORE:
-5 -3 0 3 5 7

HUNGER AFTER:
-5 -3 0 3 5 7

SNACK	
MOOD:	THOUGHTS/CHALLENGES:

HUNGER BEFORE:
-5 -3 0 3 5 7

HUNGER AFTER:
-5 -3 0 3 5 7

DINNER	
MOOD:	THOUGHTS/CHALLENGES:

HUNGER BEFORE:
-5 -3 0 3 5 7

HUNGER AFTER:
-5 -3 0 3 5 7

Hunger Rating

−5 = STARVING. You want to devour the first thing you see and have a hard time slowing down.

−3 = OVERLY HUNGRY AND IRRITABLE. You feel like you waited too long to eat.

0 = MILD TO MODERATE HUNGER. You may have physical symptoms of hunger, like a growling tummy and that "I need to eat soon" feeling, but you aren't starving or experiencing any unpleasant symptoms such as a headache or shaking.

3 = HUNGER BUT NOT CRAVING FREE. You're full, but you don't feel quite satisfied; your thoughts are still focused on food.

5 = JUST RIGHT. Your hunger is gone, and you feel satisfied. Your mind is off food, and you're ready to take on the next task. You feel energized.

7 = A LITTLE TOO MUCH. You think you overdid it. Your tummy feels stretched and uncomfortable. You feel kind of sluggish.

THE FOUR-DAY ANTI-BLOAT MENU, DAY 4

DATE:

BREAKFAST	
❏ 1 packet instant Cream of Wheat®	**MIND TRICK:**
❏ 1 cup skim milk	
❏ ¼ cup roasted or raw unsalted sunflower seeds	
❏ 2 dried plums	
❏ Glass of Sassy Water	

LUNCH	
❏ 4 oz organic deli turkey, rolled up	**MIND TRICK:**
❏ 1 cup steamed baby carrots	
❏ 1 low-fat string cheese	
❏ Glass of Sassy Water	

SNACK	
❏ Strawberry Smoothie: Blend 1 cup skim milk and 1 cup frozen unsweetened strawberries in blender for 1 minute. Transfer to glass and stir in 1 Tbsp cold-pressed organic flaxseed oil, or serve with 1 Tbsp sunflower or pumpkin seeds.	**MIND TRICK:**

DINNER	
❏ 1 cup yellow squash sautéed with 1 tsp olive oil	**MIND TRICK:**
❏ 3 oz grilled chicken breast	
❏ ½ cup cooked brown rice	
❏ Glass of Sassy Water	

JOURNAL, DAY 4

DATE: _____

BREAKFAST	
MOOD:	THOUGHTS/CHALLENGES:
HUNGER BEFORE: -5 -3 0 3 5 7	HUNGER AFTER: -5 -3 0 3 5 7

LUNCH	
MOOD:	THOUGHTS/CHALLENGES:
HUNGER BEFORE: -5 -3 0 3 5 7	HUNGER AFTER: -5 -3 0 3 5 7

SNACK	
MOOD:	THOUGHTS/CHALLENGES:
HUNGER BEFORE: -5 -3 0 3 5 7	HUNGER AFTER: -5 -3 0 3 5 7

DINNER	
MOOD:	THOUGHTS/CHALLENGES:
HUNGER BEFORE: -5 -3 0 3 5 7	HUNGER AFTER: -5 -3 0 3 5 7

Hunger Rating

–5 = STARVING. You want to devour the first thing you see and have a hard time slowing down.

–3 = OVERLY HUNGRY AND IRRITABLE. You feel like you waited too long to eat.

0 = MILD TO MODERATE HUNGER. You may have physical symptoms of hunger, like a growling tummy and that "I need to eat soon" feeling, but you aren't starving or experiencing any unpleasant symptoms such as a headache or shaking.

3 = HUNGER BUT NOT CRAVING FREE. You're full, but you don't feel quite satisfied; your thoughts are still focused on food.

5 = JUST RIGHT. Your hunger is gone, and you feel satisfied. Your mind is off food, and you're ready to take on the next task. You feel energized.

7 = A LITTLE TOO MUCH. You think you overdid it. Your tummy feels stretched and uncomfortable. You feel kind of sluggish.

DAY 1

BREAKFAST

WHAT I ATE:

MUFA: CALORIES:

TIME: HUNGER BEFORE: -5 -3 0 3 5 7   HUNGER AFTER: -5 -3 0 3 5 7

LUNCH

WHAT I ATE:

MUFA: CALORIES:

TIME: HUNGER BEFORE: -5 -3 0 3 5 7   HUNGER AFTER: -5 -3 0 3 5 7

SNACK

WHAT I ATE:

MUFA: CALORIES:

TIME: HUNGER BEFORE: -5 -3 0 3 5 7   HUNGER AFTER: -5 -3 0 3 5 7

DINNER

WHAT I ATE:

MUFA: CALORIES:

TIME: HUNGER BEFORE: -5 -3 0 3 5 7   HUNGER AFTER: -5 -3 0 3 5 7

CORE CONFIDENCE:

_____

_____

_____

_____

_____

_____

_____

_____

_____

_____

_____

_____

_____

_____

_____

_____

WORKOUT	
WALKING	Fat Blast Walk _____minutes	Calorie Torch Walk _____minutes
STRENGTH TRAINING	The Belly Routine ____sets____reps	The Metabolism Boost ___sets___reps

HOW I FELT:

DAY 2

BREAKFAST

WHAT I ATE:

MUFA: CALORIES:

TIME: HUNGER BEFORE: -5 -3 0 3 5 7   HUNGER AFTER: -5 -3 0 3 5 7

LUNCH

WHAT I ATE:

MUFA: CALORIES:

TIME: HUNGER BEFORE: -5 -3 0 3 5 7   HUNGER AFTER: -5 -3 0 3 5 7

SNACK

WHAT I ATE:

MUFA: CALORIES:

TIME: HUNGER BEFORE: -5 -3 0 3 5 7   HUNGER AFTER: -5 -3 0 3 5 7

DINNER

WHAT I ATE:

MUFA: CALORIES:

TIME: HUNGER BEFORE: -5 -3 0 3 5 7   HUNGER AFTER: -5 -3 0 3 5 7

CORE CONFIDENCE:

_____

_____

_____

_____

_____

_____

_____

_____

_____

_____

_____

_____

_____

_____

_____

_____

WORKOUT		
WALKING	Fat Blast Walk _____minutes	Calorie Torch Walk _____minutes
STRENGTH TRAINING	The Belly Routine ____sets____reps	The Metabolism Boost ___sets___reps
HOW I FELT:		

DAY 3

BREAKFAST

WHAT I ATE:

MUFA: CALORIES:

TIME: | HUNGER BEFORE: -5 -3 0 3 5 7 | HUNGER AFTER: -5 -3 0 3 5 7

LUNCH

WHAT I ATE:

MUFA: CALORIES:

TIME: | HUNGER BEFORE: -5 -3 0 3 5 7 | HUNGER AFTER: -5 -3 0 3 5 7

SNACK

WHAT I ATE:

MUFA: CALORIES:

TIME: | HUNGER BEFORE: -5 -3 0 3 5 7 | HUNGER AFTER: -5 -3 0 3 5 7

DINNER

WHAT I ATE:

MUFA: CALORIES:

TIME: | HUNGER BEFORE: -5 -3 0 3 5 7 | HUNGER AFTER: -5 -3 0 3 5 7

CORE CONFIDENCE:

_____

_____

_____

_____

_____

_____

_____

_____

_____

_____

_____

_____

_____

_____

_____

_____

_____

_____

WORKOUT		
WALKING	Fat Blast Walk _____minutes	Calorie Torch Walk _____minutes
STRENGTH TRAINING	The Belly Routine ____sets____reps	The Metabolism Boost ___sets___reps
HOW I FELT:		

DAY 4

BREAKFAST

WHAT I ATE:

MUFA: CALORIES:

TIME: HUNGER BEFORE: -5 -3 0 3 5 7   HUNGER AFTER: -5 -3 0 3 5 7

LUNCH

WHAT I ATE:

MUFA: CALORIES:

TIME: HUNGER BEFORE: -5 -3 0 3 5 7   HUNGER AFTER: -5 -3 0 3 5 7

SNACK

WHAT I ATE:

MUFA: CALORIES:

TIME: HUNGER BEFORE: -5 -3 0 3 5 7   HUNGER AFTER: -5 -3 0 3 5 7

DINNER

WHAT I ATE:

MUFA: CALORIES:

TIME: HUNGER BEFORE: -5 -3 0 3 5 7   HUNGER AFTER: -5 -3 0 3 5 7

▨ CORE CONFIDENCE:

_____

_____

_____

_____

_____

_____

_____

_____

_____

_____

_____

_____

_____

_____

_____

_____

_____

_____

WORKOUT

WALKING	Fat Blast Walk _____minutes	Calorie Torch Walk _____minutes
STRENGTH TRAINING	The Belly Routine ____sets____reps	The Metabolism Boost ___sets___reps

HOW I FELT:

DAY 5

BREAKFAST

WHAT I ATE:

MUFA: CALORIES:

TIME: HUNGER BEFORE: -5 -3 0 3 5 7 | HUNGER AFTER: -5 -3 0 3 5 7

LUNCH

WHAT I ATE:

MUFA: CALORIES:

TIME: HUNGER BEFORE: -5 -3 0 3 5 7 | HUNGER AFTER: -5 -3 0 3 5 7

SNACK

WHAT I ATE:

MUFA: CALORIES:

TIME: HUNGER BEFORE: -5 -3 0 3 5 7 | HUNGER AFTER: -5 -3 0 3 5 7

DINNER

WHAT I ATE:

MUFA: CALORIES:

TIME: HUNGER BEFORE: -5 -3 0 3 5 7 | HUNGER AFTER: -5 -3 0 3 5 7

CORE CONFIDENCE:

_____
_____
_____
_____
_____
_____
_____
_____
_____
_____
_____
_____
_____
_____
_____
_____
_____
_____

WORKOUT		
WALKING	Fat Blast Walk _____minutes	Calorie Torch Walk _____minutes
STRENGTH TRAINING	The Belly Routine ____sets____reps	The Metabolism Boost ___sets___reps
HOW I FELT:		

DAY 6

BREAKFAST

WHAT I ATE:

MUFA: CALORIES:

TIME: | HUNGER BEFORE: -5 -3 0 3 5 7 | HUNGER AFTER: -5 -3 0 3 5 7

LUNCH

WHAT I ATE:

MUFA: CALORIES:

TIME: | HUNGER BEFORE: -5 -3 0 3 5 7 | HUNGER AFTER: -5 -3 0 3 5 7

SNACK

WHAT I ATE:

MUFA: CALORIES:

TIME: | HUNGER BEFORE: -5 -3 0 3 5 7 | HUNGER AFTER: -5 -3 0 3 5 7

DINNER

WHAT I ATE:

MUFA: CALORIES:

TIME: | HUNGER BEFORE: -5 -3 0 3 5 7 | HUNGER AFTER: -5 -3 0 3 5 7

CORE CONFIDENCE:

_____

_____

_____

_____

_____

_____

_____

_____

_____

_____

_____

_____

_____

_____

_____

_____

_____

_____

WORKOUT	
WALKING	Fat Blast Walk _____minutes	Calorie Torch Walk _____minutes
STRENGTH TRAINING	The Belly Routine ____sets____reps	The Metabolism Boost ___sets___reps

HOW I FELT:

DAY 7

BREAKFAST

WHAT I ATE:

MUFA: CALORIES:

TIME: HUNGER BEFORE: -5 -3 0 3 5 7   HUNGER AFTER: -5 -3 0 3 5 7

LUNCH

WHAT I ATE:

MUFA: CALORIES:

TIME: HUNGER BEFORE: -5 -3 0 3 5 7   HUNGER AFTER: -5 -3 0 3 5 7

SNACK

WHAT I ATE:

MUFA: CALORIES:

TIME: HUNGER BEFORE: -5 -3 0 3 5 7   HUNGER AFTER: -5 -3 0 3 5 7

DINNER

WHAT I ATE:

MUFA: CALORIES:

TIME: HUNGER BEFORE: -5 -3 0 3 5 7   HUNGER AFTER: -5 -3 0 3 5 7

CORE CONFIDENCE:

_____

_____

_____

_____

_____

_____

_____

_____

_____

_____

_____

_____

_____

_____

_____

_____

WORKOUT		
WALKING	Fat Blast Walk _____minutes	Calorie Torch Walk _____minutes
STRENGTH TRAINING	The Belly Routine ____sets____reps	The Metabolism Boost ___sets___reps
HOW I FELT:		

DAY 8

BREAKFAST

WHAT I ATE:

MUFA: CALORIES:

| TIME: | HUNGER BEFORE: -5 -3 0 3 5 7 | HUNGER AFTER: -5 -3 0 3 5 7 |

LUNCH

WHAT I ATE:

MUFA: CALORIES:

| TIME: | HUNGER BEFORE: -5 -3 0 3 5 7 | HUNGER AFTER: -5 -3 0 3 5 7 |

SNACK

WHAT I ATE:

MUFA: CALORIES:

| TIME: | HUNGER BEFORE: -5 -3 0 3 5 7 | HUNGER AFTER: -5 -3 0 3 5 7 |

DINNER

WHAT I ATE:

MUFA: CALORIES:

| TIME: | HUNGER BEFORE: -5 -3 0 3 5 7 | HUNGER AFTER: -5 -3 0 3 5 7 |

CORE CONFIDENCE:

_____

_____

_____

_____

_____

_____

_____

_____

_____

_____

_____

_____

_____

_____

_____

_____

WORKOUT		
WALKING	Fat Blast Walk _____minutes	Calorie Torch Walk _____minutes
STRENGTH TRAINING	The Belly Routine ____sets____reps	The Metabolism Boost ___sets___reps
HOW I FELT:		

DAY 9

BREAKFAST

WHAT I ATE:

MUFA: CALORIES:

TIME: HUNGER BEFORE: -5 -3 0 3 5 7   HUNGER AFTER: -5 -3 0 3 5 7

LUNCH

WHAT I ATE:

MUFA: CALORIES:

TIME: HUNGER BEFORE: -5 -3 0 3 5 7   HUNGER AFTER: -5 -3 0 3 5 7

SNACK

WHAT I ATE:

MUFA: CALORIES:

TIME: HUNGER BEFORE: -5 -3 0 3 5 7   HUNGER AFTER: -5 -3 0 3 5 7

DINNER

WHAT I ATE:

MUFA: CALORIES:

TIME: HUNGER BEFORE: -5 -3 0 3 5 7   HUNGER AFTER: -5 -3 0 3 5 7

CORE CONFIDENCE:

_____

_____

_____

_____

_____

_____

_____

_____

_____

_____

_____

_____

_____

_____

_____

_____

_____

_____

WORKOUT	
WALKING	Fat Blast Walk _____minutes	Calorie Torch Walk _____minutes
STRENGTH TRAINING	The Belly Routine ____sets____reps	The Metabolism Boost ___sets___reps

HOW I FELT:

DAY 10

BREAKFAST

WHAT I ATE:

MUFA: CALORIES:

TIME: HUNGER BEFORE: -5 -3 0 3 5 7   HUNGER AFTER: -5 -3 0 3 5 7

LUNCH

WHAT I ATE:

MUFA: CALORIES:

TIME: HUNGER BEFORE: -5 -3 0 3 5 7   HUNGER AFTER: -5 -3 0 3 5 7

SNACK

WHAT I ATE:

MUFA: CALORIES:

TIME: HUNGER BEFORE: -5 -3 0 3 5 7   HUNGER AFTER: -5 -3 0 3 5 7

DINNER

WHAT I ATE:

MUFA: CALORIES:

TIME: HUNGER BEFORE: -5 -3 0 3 5 7   HUNGER AFTER: -5 -3 0 3 5 7

CORE CONFIDENCE:

_____

_____

_____

_____

_____

_____

_____

_____

_____

_____

_____

_____

_____

_____

_____

WORKOUT		
WALKING	Fat Blast Walk _____minutes	Calorie Torch Walk _____minutes
STRENGTH TRAINING	The Belly Routine ____sets____reps	The Metabolism Boost ___sets___reps
HOW I FELT:		

DAY 11

BREAKFAST

WHAT I ATE:

MUFA: CALORIES:

TIME: | HUNGER BEFORE: -5 -3 0 3 5 7 | HUNGER AFTER: -5 -3 0 3 5 7

LUNCH

WHAT I ATE:

MUFA: CALORIES:

TIME: | HUNGER BEFORE: -5 -3 0 3 5 7 | HUNGER AFTER: -5 -3 0 3 5 7

SNACK

WHAT I ATE:

MUFA: CALORIES:

TIME: | HUNGER BEFORE: -5 -3 0 3 5 7 | HUNGER AFTER: -5 -3 0 3 5 7

DINNER

WHAT I ATE:

MUFA: CALORIES:

TIME: | HUNGER BEFORE: -5 -3 0 3 5 7 | HUNGER AFTER: -5 -3 0 3 5 7

■ CORE CONFIDENCE:

_____

_____

_____

_____

_____

_____

_____

_____

_____

_____

_____

_____

_____

_____

_____

_____

_____

WORKOUT	
WALKING	Fat Blast Walk _____minutes	Calorie Torch Walk _____minutes
STRENGTH TRAINING	The Belly Routine ____sets____reps	The Metabolism Boost ___sets___reps

HOW I FELT:

DAY 12

BREAKFAST

WHAT I ATE:

MUFA: CALORIES:

TIME: HUNGER BEFORE: -5 -3 0 3 5 7   HUNGER AFTER: -5 -3 0 3 5 7

LUNCH

WHAT I ATE:

MUFA: CALORIES:

TIME: HUNGER BEFORE: -5 -3 0 3 5 7   HUNGER AFTER: -5 -3 0 3 5 7

SNACK

WHAT I ATE:

MUFA: CALORIES:

TIME: HUNGER BEFORE: -5 -3 0 3 5 7   HUNGER AFTER: -5 -3 0 3 5 7

DINNER

WHAT I ATE:

MUFA: CALORIES:

TIME: HUNGER BEFORE: -5 -3 0 3 5 7   HUNGER AFTER: -5 -3 0 3 5 7

CORE CONFIDENCE:

_____

_____

_____

_____

_____

_____

_____

_____

_____

_____

_____

_____

_____

_____

_____

_____

WORKOUT		
WALKING	Fat Blast Walk _____ minutes	Calorie Torch Walk _____ minutes
STRENGTH TRAINING	The Belly Routine ____ sets ____ reps	The Metabolism Boost ___ sets ___ reps
HOW I FELT:		

DAY 13

BREAKFAST

WHAT I ATE:

MUFA: CALORIES:

TIME: HUNGER BEFORE: -5 -3 0 3 5 7 | HUNGER AFTER: -5 -3 0 3 5 7

LUNCH

WHAT I ATE:

MUFA: CALORIES:

TIME: HUNGER BEFORE: -5 -3 0 3 5 7 | HUNGER AFTER: -5 -3 0 3 5 7

SNACK

WHAT I ATE:

MUFA: CALORIES:

TIME: HUNGER BEFORE: -5 -3 0 3 5 7 | HUNGER AFTER: -5 -3 0 3 5 7

DINNER

WHAT I ATE:

MUFA: CALORIES:

TIME: HUNGER BEFORE: -5 -3 0 3 5 7 | HUNGER AFTER: -5 -3 0 3 5 7

CORE CONFIDENCE:

_____

_____

_____

_____

_____

_____

_____

_____

_____

_____

_____

_____

_____

_____

_____

_____

_____

_____

WORKOUT		
WALKING	Fat Blast Walk _____minutes	Calorie Torch Walk _____minutes
STRENGTH TRAINING	The Belly Routine ____sets____reps	The Metabolism Boost ___sets___reps
HOW I FELT:		

DAY 14

BREAKFAST

WHAT I ATE:

MUFA: CALORIES:

| TIME: | HUNGER BEFORE: -5 -3 0 3 5 7 | HUNGER AFTER: -5 -3 0 3 5 7 |

LUNCH

WHAT I ATE:

MUFA: CALORIES:

| TIME: | HUNGER BEFORE: -5 -3 0 3 5 7 | HUNGER AFTER: -5 -3 0 3 5 7 |

SNACK

WHAT I ATE:

MUFA: CALORIES:

| TIME: | HUNGER BEFORE: -5 -3 0 3 5 7 | HUNGER AFTER: -5 -3 0 3 5 7 |

DINNER

WHAT I ATE:

MUFA: CALORIES:

| TIME: | HUNGER BEFORE: -5 -3 0 3 5 7 | HUNGER AFTER: -5 -3 0 3 5 7 |

CORE CONFIDENCE:

_____

_____

_____

_____

_____

_____

_____

_____

_____

_____

_____

_____

_____

_____

_____

_____

WORKOUT		
WALKING	Fat Blast Walk _____ minutes	Calorie Torch Walk _____ minutes
STRENGTH TRAINING	The Belly Routine ____sets____reps	The Metabolism Boost ___sets___reps
HOW I FELT:		

DAY 15

BREAKFAST

WHAT I ATE:

MUFA: CALORIES:

TIME: | HUNGER BEFORE: -5 -3 0 3 5 7 | HUNGER AFTER: -5 -3 0 3 5 7

LUNCH

WHAT I ATE:

MUFA: CALORIES:

TIME: | HUNGER BEFORE: -5 -3 0 3 5 7 | HUNGER AFTER: -5 -3 0 3 5 7

SNACK

WHAT I ATE:

MUFA: CALORIES:

TIME: | HUNGER BEFORE: -5 -3 0 3 5 7 | HUNGER AFTER: -5 -3 0 3 5 7

DINNER

WHAT I ATE:

MUFA: CALORIES:

TIME: | HUNGER BEFORE: -5 -3 0 3 5 7 | HUNGER AFTER: -5 -3 0 3 5 7

CORE CONFIDENCE:

_____

_____

_____

_____

_____

_____

_____

_____

_____

_____

_____

_____

_____

_____

_____

_____

WORKOUT		
WALKING	Fat Blast Walk _____minutes	Calorie Torch Walk _____minutes
STRENGTH TRAINING	The Belly Routine ____sets____reps	The Metabolism Boost ___sets___reps
HOW I FELT:		

DAY 16

BREAKFAST

WHAT I ATE:

MUFA: CALORIES:

TIME: HUNGER BEFORE: -5 -3 0 3 5 7   HUNGER AFTER: -5 -3 0 3 5 7

LUNCH

WHAT I ATE:

MUFA: CALORIES:

TIME: HUNGER BEFORE: -5 -3 0 3 5 7   HUNGER AFTER: -5 -3 0 3 5 7

SNACK

WHAT I ATE:

MUFA: CALORIES:

TIME: HUNGER BEFORE: -5 -3 0 3 5 7   HUNGER AFTER: -5 -3 0 3 5 7

DINNER

WHAT I ATE:

MUFA: CALORIES:

TIME: HUNGER BEFORE: -5 -3 0 3 5 7   HUNGER AFTER: -5 -3 0 3 5 7

CORE CONFIDENCE:

_____

_____

_____

_____

_____

_____

_____

_____

_____

_____

_____

_____

_____

_____

_____

_____

_____

WORKOUT		
WALKING	Fat Blast Walk _____minutes	Calorie Torch Walk _____minutes
STRENGTH TRAINING	The Belly Routine ____sets____reps	The Metabolism Boost ___sets___reps
HOW I FELT:		

DAY 17

BREAKFAST

WHAT I ATE:

MUFA: CALORIES:

TIME: | HUNGER BEFORE: -5 -3 0 3 5 7 | HUNGER AFTER: -5 -3 0 3 5 7

LUNCH

WHAT I ATE:

MUFA: CALORIES:

TIME: | HUNGER BEFORE: -5 -3 0 3 5 7 | HUNGER AFTER: -5 -3 0 3 5 7

SNACK

WHAT I ATE:

MUFA: CALORIES:

TIME: | HUNGER BEFORE: -5 -3 0 3 5 7 | HUNGER AFTER: -5 -3 0 3 5 7

DINNER

WHAT I ATE:

MUFA: CALORIES:

TIME: | HUNGER BEFORE: -5 -3 0 3 5 7 | HUNGER AFTER: -5 -3 0 3 5 7

CORE CONFIDENCE:

_____

_____

_____

_____

_____

_____

_____

_____

_____

_____

_____

_____

_____

_____

_____

_____

_____

_____

_____

WORKOUT	
WALKING	Fat Blast Walk _____minutes	Calorie Torch Walk _____minutes
STRENGTH TRAINING	The Belly Routine ____sets____reps	The Metabolism Boost ___sets___reps
HOW I FELT:	

DAY 18

BREAKFAST

WHAT I ATE:

MUFA: CALORIES:

TIME: HUNGER BEFORE: -5 -3 0 3 5 7   HUNGER AFTER: -5 -3 0 3 5 7

LUNCH

WHAT I ATE:

MUFA: CALORIES:

TIME: HUNGER BEFORE: -5 -3 0 3 5 7   HUNGER AFTER: -5 -3 0 3 5 7

SNACK

WHAT I ATE:

MUFA: CALORIES:

TIME: HUNGER BEFORE: -5 -3 0 3 5 7   HUNGER AFTER: -5 -3 0 3 5 7

DINNER

WHAT I ATE:

MUFA: CALORIES:

TIME: HUNGER BEFORE: -5 -3 0 3 5 7   HUNGER AFTER: -5 -3 0 3 5 7

CORE CONFIDENCE:

_____

_____

_____

_____

_____

_____

_____

_____

_____

_____

_____

_____

_____

_____

_____

_____

_____

_____

WORKOUT		
WALKING	Fat Blast Walk _____minutes	Calorie Torch Walk _____minutes
STRENGTH TRAINING	The Belly Routine ____sets____reps	The Metabolism Boost ___sets___reps
HOW I FELT:		

DAY 19

BREAKFAST

WHAT I ATE:

MUFA: CALORIES:

TIME: | HUNGER BEFORE: -5 -3 0 3 5 7 | HUNGER AFTER: -5 -3 0 3 5 7

LUNCH

WHAT I ATE:

MUFA: CALORIES:

TIME: | HUNGER BEFORE: -5 -3 0 3 5 7 | HUNGER AFTER: -5 -3 0 3 5 7

SNACK

WHAT I ATE:

MUFA: CALORIES:

TIME: | HUNGER BEFORE: -5 -3 0 3 5 7 | HUNGER AFTER: -5 -3 0 3 5 7

DINNER

WHAT I ATE:

MUFA: CALORIES:

TIME: | HUNGER BEFORE: -5 -3 0 3 5 7 | HUNGER AFTER: -5 -3 0 3 5 7

CORE CONFIDENCE:

_____

_____

_____

_____

_____

_____

_____

_____

_____

_____

_____

_____

_____

_____

_____

_____

_____

WORKOUT		
WALKING	Fat Blast Walk _____minutes	Calorie Torch Walk _____minutes
STRENGTH TRAINING	The Belly Routine ____sets____reps	The Metabolism Boost ___sets___reps

HOW I FELT:

DAY 20

BREAKFAST

WHAT I ATE:

MUFA: CALORIES:

TIME: | HUNGER BEFORE: -5 -3 0 3 5 7 | HUNGER AFTER: -5 -3 0 3 5 7

LUNCH

WHAT I ATE:

MUFA: CALORIES:

TIME: | HUNGER BEFORE: -5 -3 0 3 5 7 | HUNGER AFTER: -5 -3 0 3 5 7

SNACK

WHAT I ATE:

MUFA: CALORIES:

TIME: | HUNGER BEFORE: -5 -3 0 3 5 7 | HUNGER AFTER: -5 -3 0 3 5 7

DINNER

WHAT I ATE:

MUFA: CALORIES:

TIME: | HUNGER BEFORE: -5 -3 0 3 5 7 | HUNGER AFTER: -5 -3 0 3 5 7

▨ CORE CONFIDENCE:

_____

_____

_____

_____

_____

_____

_____

_____

_____

_____

_____

_____

_____

_____

_____

_____

_____

WORKOUT		
WALKING	Fat Blast Walk _____minutes	Calorie Torch Walk _____minutes
STRENGTH TRAINING	The Belly Routine ____sets____reps	The Metabolism Boost ___sets___reps
HOW I FELT:		

DAY 21

BREAKFAST

WHAT I ATE:

MUFA: CALORIES:

TIME:	HUNGER BEFORE: -5 -3 0 3 5 7	HUNGER AFTER: -5 -3 0 3 5 7

LUNCH

WHAT I ATE:

MUFA: CALORIES:

TIME:	HUNGER BEFORE: -5 -3 0 3 5 7	HUNGER AFTER: -5 -3 0 3 5 7

SNACK

WHAT I ATE:

MUFA: CALORIES:

TIME:	HUNGER BEFORE: -5 -3 0 3 5 7	HUNGER AFTER: -5 -3 0 3 5 7

DINNER

WHAT I ATE:

MUFA: CALORIES:

TIME:	HUNGER BEFORE: -5 -3 0 3 5 7	HUNGER AFTER: -5 -3 0 3 5 7

CORE CONFIDENCE:

_____
_____
_____
_____
_____
_____
_____
_____
_____
_____
_____
_____
_____
_____
_____
_____
_____

WORKOUT	
WALKING	Fat Blast Walk _____minutes	Calorie Torch Walk _____minutes
STRENGTH TRAINING	The Belly Routine ____sets____reps	The Metabolism Boost ___sets___reps

HOW I FELT:

DAY 22

BREAKFAST

WHAT I ATE:

MUFA: CALORIES:

TIME: HUNGER BEFORE: -5 -3 0 3 5 7   HUNGER AFTER: -5 -3 0 3 5 7

LUNCH

WHAT I ATE:

MUFA: CALORIES:

TIME: HUNGER BEFORE: -5 -3 0 3 5 7   HUNGER AFTER: -5 -3 0 3 5 7

SNACK

WHAT I ATE:

MUFA: CALORIES:

TIME: HUNGER BEFORE: -5 -3 0 3 5 7   HUNGER AFTER: -5 -3 0 3 5 7

DINNER

WHAT I ATE:

MUFA: CALORIES:

TIME: HUNGER BEFORE: -5 -3 0 3 5 7   HUNGER AFTER: -5 -3 0 3 5 7

CORE CONFIDENCE:

WORKOUT

WALKING	Fat Blast Walk _____minutes	Calorie Torch Walk _____minutes
STRENGTH TRAINING	The Belly Routine ____sets____reps	The Metabolism Boost ___sets___reps

HOW I FELT:

DAY 23

BREAKFAST

WHAT I ATE:

MUFA: CALORIES:

TIME: | HUNGER BEFORE: -5 -3 0 3 5 7 | HUNGER AFTER: -5 -3 0 3 5 7

LUNCH

WHAT I ATE:

MUFA: CALORIES:

TIME: | HUNGER BEFORE: -5 -3 0 3 5 7 | HUNGER AFTER: -5 -3 0 3 5 7

SNACK

WHAT I ATE:

MUFA: CALORIES:

TIME: | HUNGER BEFORE: -5 -3 0 3 5 7 | HUNGER AFTER: -5 -3 0 3 5 7

DINNER

WHAT I ATE:

MUFA: CALORIES:

TIME: | HUNGER BEFORE: -5 -3 0 3 5 7 | HUNGER AFTER: -5 -3 0 3 5 7

▨ CORE CONFIDENCE:

_____

_____

_____

_____

_____

_____

_____

_____

_____

_____

_____

_____

_____

_____

_____

_____

WORKOUT		
WALKING	Fat Blast Walk _____minutes	Calorie Torch Walk _____minutes
STRENGTH TRAINING	The Belly Routine ____sets____reps	The Metabolism Boost ___sets___reps

HOW I FELT:

DAY 24

BREAKFAST

WHAT I ATE:

MUFA: CALORIES:

TIME: HUNGER BEFORE: -5 -3 0 3 5 7   HUNGER AFTER: -5 -3 0 3 5 7

LUNCH

WHAT I ATE:

MUFA: CALORIES:

TIME: HUNGER BEFORE: -5 -3 0 3 5 7   HUNGER AFTER: -5 -3 0 3 5 7

SNACK

WHAT I ATE:

MUFA: CALORIES:

TIME: HUNGER BEFORE: -5 -3 0 3 5 7   HUNGER AFTER: -5 -3 0 3 5 7

DINNER

WHAT I ATE:

MUFA: CALORIES:

TIME: HUNGER BEFORE: -5 -3 0 3 5 7   HUNGER AFTER: -5 -3 0 3 5 7

CORE CONFIDENCE:

_____

_____

_____

_____

_____

_____

_____

_____

_____

_____

_____

_____

_____

_____

_____

_____

_____

_____

WORKOUT		
WALKING	Fat Blast Walk _____minutes	Calorie Torch Walk _____minutes
STRENGTH TRAINING	The Belly Routine ____sets____reps	The Metabolism Boost ___sets___reps

HOW I FELT:

DAY 25

BREAKFAST

WHAT I ATE:

MUFA: CALORIES:

TIME: HUNGER BEFORE: -5 -3 0 3 5 7   HUNGER AFTER: -5 -3 0 3 5 7

LUNCH

WHAT I ATE:

MUFA: CALORIES:

TIME: HUNGER BEFORE: -5 -3 0 3 5 7   HUNGER AFTER: -5 -3 0 3 5 7

SNACK

WHAT I ATE:

MUFA: CALORIES:

TIME: HUNGER BEFORE: -5 -3 0 3 5 7   HUNGER AFTER: -5 -3 0 3 5 7

DINNER

WHAT I ATE:

MUFA: CALORIES:

TIME: HUNGER BEFORE: -5 -3 0 3 5 7   HUNGER AFTER: -5 -3 0 3 5 7

CORE CONFIDENCE:

WORKOUT

WALKING	Fat Blast Walk _____minutes	Calorie Torch Walk _____minutes
STRENGTH TRAINING	The Belly Routine ____sets____reps	The Metabolism Boost ___sets___reps
HOW I FELT:		

DAY 26

BREAKFAST

WHAT I ATE:

MUFA: CALORIES:

TIME: | HUNGER BEFORE: -5 -3 0 3 5 7 | HUNGER AFTER: -5 -3 0 3 5 7

LUNCH

WHAT I ATE:

MUFA: CALORIES:

TIME: | HUNGER BEFORE: -5 -3 0 3 5 7 | HUNGER AFTER: -5 -3 0 3 5 7

SNACK

WHAT I ATE:

MUFA: CALORIES:

TIME: | HUNGER BEFORE: -5 -3 0 3 5 7 | HUNGER AFTER: -5 -3 0 3 5 7

DINNER

WHAT I ATE:

MUFA: CALORIES:

TIME: | HUNGER BEFORE: -5 -3 0 3 5 7 | HUNGER AFTER: -5 -3 0 3 5 7

CORE CONFIDENCE:

_____

_____

_____

_____

_____

_____

_____

_____

_____

_____

_____

_____

_____

_____

_____

_____

WORKOUT	
WALKING	Fat Blast Walk _____minutes	Calorie Torch Walk _____minutes
STRENGTH TRAINING	The Belly Routine ____sets____reps	The Metabolism Boost ___sets___reps
HOW I FELT:		

DAY 27

BREAKFAST

WHAT I ATE:

MUFA: CALORIES:

TIME: HUNGER BEFORE: -5 -3 0 3 5 7 | HUNGER AFTER: -5 -3 0 3 5 7

LUNCH

WHAT I ATE:

MUFA: CALORIES:

TIME: HUNGER BEFORE: -5 -3 0 3 5 7 | HUNGER AFTER: -5 -3 0 3 5 7

SNACK

WHAT I ATE:

MUFA: CALORIES:

TIME: HUNGER BEFORE: -5 -3 0 3 5 7 | HUNGER AFTER: -5 -3 0 3 5 7

DINNER

WHAT I ATE:

MUFA: CALORIES:

TIME: HUNGER BEFORE: -5 -3 0 3 5 7 | HUNGER AFTER: -5 -3 0 3 5 7

CORE CONFIDENCE:

_____

_____

_____

_____

_____

_____

_____

_____

_____

_____

_____

_____

_____

_____

_____

_____

WORKOUT	
WALKING	Fat Blast Walk _____minutes	Calorie Torch Walk _____minutes
STRENGTH TRAINING	The Belly Routine ____sets____reps	The Metabolism Boost ___sets___reps

HOW I FELT:

DAY 28

BREAKFAST

WHAT I ATE:

MUFA: CALORIES:

TIME: HUNGER BEFORE: -5 -3 0 3 5 7   HUNGER AFTER: -5 -3 0 3 5 7

LUNCH

WHAT I ATE:

MUFA: CALORIES:

TIME: HUNGER BEFORE: -5 -3 0 3 5 7   HUNGER AFTER: -5 -3 0 3 5 7

SNACK

WHAT I ATE:

MUFA: CALORIES:

TIME: HUNGER BEFORE: -5 -3 0 3 5 7   HUNGER AFTER: -5 -3 0 3 5 7

DINNER

WHAT I ATE:

MUFA: CALORIES:

TIME: HUNGER BEFORE: -5 -3 0 3 5 7   HUNGER AFTER: -5 -3 0 3 5 7

▧ CORE CONFIDENCE:

_____

_____

_____

_____

_____

_____

_____

_____

_____

_____

_____

_____

_____

_____

_____

_____

_____

_____

WORKOUT	
WALKING	Fat Blast Walk _____minutes	Calorie Torch Walk _____minutes
STRENGTH TRAINING	The Belly Routine ____sets____reps	The Metabolism Boost ___sets___reps
HOW I FELT:		

THE FOUR-DAY ANTI-BLOAT MENU, DAY 1

DATE:

BREAKFAST	
❑ 1 cup unsweetened cornflakes	**MIND TRICK:**
❑ 1 cup skim milk	
❑ ½ cup unsweetened applesauce	
❑ ¼ cup roasted or raw unsalted sunflower seeds	
❑ Glass of Sassy Water	

LUNCH	
❑ 4 oz organic deli turkey, rolled up	**MIND TRICK:**
❑ 1 low-fat string cheese	
❑ 1 pint fresh grape tomatoes	
❑ Glass of Sassy Water	

SNACK	
❑ Blueberry Smoothie: Blend 1 cup skim milk and 1 cup frozen unsweetened blueberries in blender for 1 minute. Transfer to glass and stir in 1 Tbsp cold-pressed organic flaxseed oil, or serve with 1 Tbsp sunflower or pumpkin seeds.	**MIND TRICK:**

DINNER	
❑ 1 cup cooked green beans	**MIND TRICK:**
❑ 4 oz grilled tilapia	
❑ ½ cup roasted red potatoes drizzled with 1 tsp olive oil	
❑ Glass of Sassy Water	

JOURNAL, DAY 1

DATE:

BREAKFAST

MOOD:

THOUGHTS/CHALLENGES:

HUNGER BEFORE:
-5 -3 0 3 5 7

HUNGER AFTER:
-5 -3 0 3 5 7

LUNCH

MOOD:

THOUGHTS/CHALLENGES:

HUNGER BEFORE:
-5 -3 0 3 5 7

HUNGER AFTER:
-5 -3 0 3 5 7

SNACK

MOOD:

THOUGHTS/CHALLENGES:

HUNGER BEFORE:
-5 -3 0 3 5 7

HUNGER AFTER:
-5 -3 0 3 5 7

DINNER

MOOD:

THOUGHTS/CHALLENGES:

HUNGER BEFORE:
-5 -3 0 3 5 7

HUNGER AFTER:
-5 -3 0 3 5 7

Hunger Rating

–5 = STARVING. You want to devour the first thing you see and have a hard time slowing down.

–3 = OVERLY HUNGRY AND IRRITABLE. You feel like you waited too long to eat.

0 = MILD TO MODERATE HUNGER. You may have physical symptoms of hunger, like a growling tummy and that "I need to eat soon" feeling, but you aren't starving or experiencing any unpleasant symptoms such as a headache or shaking.

3 = HUNGER BUT NOT CRAVING FREE. You're full, but you don't feel quite satisfied; your thoughts are still focused on food.

5 = JUST RIGHT. Your hunger is gone, and you feel satisfied. Your mind is off food, and you're ready to take on the next task. You feel energized.

7 = A LITTLE TOO MUCH. You think you overdid it. Your tummy feels stretched and uncomfortable. You feel kind of sluggish.

THE FOUR-DAY ANTI-BLOAT MENU, DAY 2

DATE:

BREAKFAST

- ❑ 1 cup unsweetened puffed rice cereal
- ❑ 1 cup skim milk
- ❑ ¼ cup roasted or raw unsalted sunflower seeds
- ❑ 4 oz pineapple tidbits canned in juice
- ❑ Glass of Sassy Water

MIND TRICK:

LUNCH

- ❑ 3 oz chunk light tuna in water
- ❑ 1 cup steamed baby carrots
- ❑ 1 low-fat string cheese
- ❑ Glass of Sassy Water

MIND TRICK:

SNACK

- ❑ Pineapple Smoothie: Blend 1 cup skim milk, 4 oz canned pineapple tidbits in juice, and a handful of ice in blender for 1 minute. Transfer to glass and stir in 1 Tbsp cold-pressed organic flaxseed oil, or serve with 1 Tbsp sunflower or pumpkin seeds.

MIND TRICK:

DINNER

- ❑ 1 cup fresh cremini mushrooms sautéed with 1 tsp olive oil
- ❑ 3 oz grilled chicken breast
- ❑ ½ cup cooked brown rice
- ❑ Glass of Sassy Water

MIND TRICK:

JOURNAL, DAY 2

DATE: _____

BREAKFAST	
MOOD:	THOUGHTS/CHALLENGES:
HUNGER BEFORE: -5 -3 0 3 5 7	HUNGER AFTER: -5 -3 0 3 5 7

LUNCH	
MOOD:	THOUGHTS/CHALLENGES:
HUNGER BEFORE: -5 -3 0 3 5 7	HUNGER AFTER: -5 -3 0 3 5 7

SNACK	
MOOD:	THOUGHTS/CHALLENGES:
HUNGER BEFORE: -5 -3 0 3 5 7	HUNGER AFTER: -5 -3 0 3 5 7

DINNER	
MOOD:	THOUGHTS/CHALLENGES:
HUNGER BEFORE: -5 -3 0 3 5 7	HUNGER AFTER: -5 -3 0 3 5 7

Hunger Rating

-5 = STARVING. You want to devour the first thing you see and have a hard time slowing down.

-3 = OVERLY HUNGRY AND IRRITABLE. You feel like you waited too long to eat.

0 = MILD TO MODERATE HUNGER. You may have physical symptoms of hunger, like a growling tummy and that "I need to eat soon" feeling, but you aren't starving or experiencing any unpleasant symptoms such as a headache or shaking.

3 = HUNGER BUT NOT CRAVING FREE. You're full, but you don't feel quite satisfied; your thoughts are still focused on food.

5 = JUST RIGHT. Your hunger is gone, and you feel satisfied. Your mind is off food, and you're ready to take on the next task. You feel energized.

7 = A LITTLE TOO MUCH. You think you overdid it. Your tummy feels stretched and uncomfortable. You feel kind of sluggish.

THE FOUR-DAY ANTI-BLOAT MENU, DAY 3

DATE:

BREAKFAST	
❑ 1 cup unsweetened cornflakes	**MIND TRICK:**
❑ 1 cup skim milk	
❑ ¼ cup roasted or raw unsalted sunflower seeds	
❑ 2 Tbsp raisins	
❑ Glass of Sassy Water	

LUNCH	
❑ 4 oz organic deli turkey, rolled up	**MIND TRICK:**
❑ 1 low-fat string cheese	
❑ 1 pint grape tomatoes	
❑ Glass of Sassy Water	

SNACK	
❑ Peach Smoothie: Blend 1 cup skim milk and 1 cup frozen unsweetened peaches in blender for 1 minute. Transfer to glass and stir in 1 Tbsp cold-pressed organic flaxseed oil, or serve with 1 Tbsp sunflower or pumpkin seeds.	**MIND TRICK:**

DINNER	
❑ 1 cup cooked green beans	**MIND TRICK:**
❑ 3 oz grilled or baked turkey breast cutlet	
❑ ½ cup roasted red potatoes drizzled with 1 tsp olive oil	
❑ Glass of Sassy Water	

JOURNAL, DAY 3

DATE: _____

BREAKFAST	
MOOD:	THOUGHTS/CHALLENGES:
HUNGER BEFORE: -5 -3 0 3 5 7	HUNGER AFTER: -5 -3 0 3 5 7

LUNCH	
MOOD:	THOUGHTS/CHALLENGES:
HUNGER BEFORE: -5 -3 0 3 5 7	HUNGER AFTER: -5 -3 0 3 5 7

SNACK	
MOOD:	THOUGHTS/CHALLENGES:
HUNGER BEFORE: -5 -3 0 3 5 7	HUNGER AFTER: -5 -3 0 3 5 7

DINNER	
MOOD:	THOUGHTS/CHALLENGES:
HUNGER BEFORE: -5 -3 0 3 5 7	HUNGER AFTER: -5 -3 0 3 5 7

Hunger Rating

-5 = STARVING. You want to devour the first thing you see and have a hard time slowing down.

-3 = OVERLY HUNGRY AND IRRITABLE. You feel like you waited too long to eat.

0 = MILD TO MODERATE HUNGER. You may have physical symptoms of hunger, like a growling tummy and that "I need to eat soon" feeling, but you aren't starving or experiencing any unpleasant symptoms such as a headache or shaking.

3 = HUNGER BUT NOT CRAVING FREE. You're full, but you don't feel quite satisfied; your thoughts are still focused on food.

5 = JUST RIGHT. Your hunger is gone, and you feel satisfied. Your mind is off food, and you're ready to take on the next task. You feel energized.

7 = A LITTLE TOO MUCH. You think you overdid it. Your tummy feels stretched and uncomfortable. You feel kind of sluggish.

THE FOUR-DAY ANTI-BLOAT MENU, DAY 4

DATE:

BREAKFAST

- ❏ 1 packet instant Cream of Wheat®
- ❏ 1 cup skim milk
- ❏ ¼ cup roasted or raw unsalted sunflower seeds
- ❏ 2 dried plums
- ❏ Glass of Sassy Water

MIND TRICK:

LUNCH

- ❏ 4 oz organic deli turkey, rolled up
- ❏ 1 cup steamed baby carrots
- ❏ 1 low-fat string cheese
- ❏ Glass of Sassy Water

MIND TRICK:

SNACK

- ❏ Strawberry Smoothie: Blend 1 cup skim milk and 1 cup frozen unsweetened strawberries in blender for 1 minute. Transfer to glass and stir in 1 Tbsp cold-pressed organic flaxseed oil, or serve with 1 Tbsp sunflower or pumpkin seeds.

MIND TRICK:

DINNER

- ❏ 1 cup yellow squash sautéed with 1 tsp olive oil
- ❏ 3 oz grilled chicken breast
- ❏ ½ cup cooked brown rice
- ❏ Glass of Sassy Water

MIND TRICK:

JOURNAL, DAY 4

DATE: _____

BREAKFAST	
MOOD:	THOUGHTS/CHALLENGES:
HUNGER BEFORE: -5 -3 0 3 5 7	HUNGER AFTER: -5 -3 0 3 5 7

LUNCH	
MOOD:	THOUGHTS/CHALLENGES:
HUNGER BEFORE: -5 -3 0 3 5 7	HUNGER AFTER: -5 -3 0 3 5 7

SNACK	
MOOD:	THOUGHTS/CHALLENGES:
HUNGER BEFORE: -5 -3 0 3 5 7	HUNGER AFTER: -5 -3 0 3 5 7

DINNER	
MOOD:	THOUGHTS/CHALLENGES:
HUNGER BEFORE: -5 -3 0 3 5 7	HUNGER AFTER: -5 -3 0 3 5 7

Hunger Rating

–5 = STARVING. You want to devour the first thing you see and have a hard time slowing down.

–3 = OVERLY HUNGRY AND IRRITABLE. You feel like you waited too long to eat.

0 = MILD TO MODERATE HUNGER. You may have physical symptoms of hunger, like a growling tummy and that "I need to eat soon" feeling, but you aren't starving or experiencing any unpleasant symptoms such as a headache or shaking.

3 = HUNGER BUT NOT CRAVING FREE. You're full, but you don't feel quite satisfied; your thoughts are still focused on food.

5 = JUST RIGHT. Your hunger is gone, and you feel satisfied. Your mind is off food, and you're ready to take on the next task. You feel energized.

7 = A LITTLE TOO MUCH. You think you overdid it. Your tummy feels stretched and uncomfortable. You feel kind of sluggish.

DAY 1

BREAKFAST

WHAT I ATE:

MUFA: CALORIES:

TIME: | HUNGER BEFORE: -5 -3 0 3 5 7 | HUNGER AFTER: -5 -3 0 3 5 7

LUNCH

WHAT I ATE:

MUFA: CALORIES:

TIME: | HUNGER BEFORE: -5 -3 0 3 5 7 | HUNGER AFTER: -5 -3 0 3 5 7

SNACK

WHAT I ATE:

MUFA: CALORIES:

TIME: | HUNGER BEFORE: -5 -3 0 3 5 7 | HUNGER AFTER: -5 -3 0 3 5 7

DINNER

WHAT I ATE:

MUFA: CALORIES:

TIME: | HUNGER BEFORE: -5 -3 0 3 5 7 | HUNGER AFTER: -5 -3 0 3 5 7

CORE CONFIDENCE:

_____

_____

_____

_____

_____

_____

_____

_____

_____

_____

_____

_____

_____

_____

_____

_____

_____

_____

WORKOUT		
WALKING	Fat Blast Walk _____minutes	Calorie Torch Walk _____minutes
STRENGTH TRAINING	The Belly Routine ____sets____reps	The Metabolism Boost ___sets___reps

HOW I FELT:

DAY 2

BREAKFAST

WHAT I ATE:

MUFA: CALORIES:

TIME: | HUNGER BEFORE: -5 -3 0 3 5 7 | HUNGER AFTER: -5 -3 0 3 5 7

LUNCH

WHAT I ATE:

MUFA: CALORIES:

TIME: | HUNGER BEFORE: -5 -3 0 3 5 7 | HUNGER AFTER: -5 -3 0 3 5 7

SNACK

WHAT I ATE:

MUFA: CALORIES:

TIME: | HUNGER BEFORE: -5 -3 0 3 5 7 | HUNGER AFTER: -5 -3 0 3 5 7

DINNER

WHAT I ATE:

MUFA: CALORIES:

TIME: | HUNGER BEFORE: -5 -3 0 3 5 7 | HUNGER AFTER: -5 -3 0 3 5 7

CORE CONFIDENCE:

	WORKOUT	
WALKING	Fat Blast Walk _____minutes	Calorie Torch Walk _____minutes
STRENGTH TRAINING	The Belly Routine ____sets____reps	The Metabolism Boost ___sets___reps

HOW I FELT:

DAY 3

BREAKFAST

WHAT I ATE:

MUFA: CALORIES:

TIME: HUNGER BEFORE: -5 -3 0 3 5 7 | HUNGER AFTER: -5 -3 0 3 5 7

LUNCH

WHAT I ATE:

MUFA: CALORIES:

TIME: HUNGER BEFORE: -5 -3 0 3 5 7 | HUNGER AFTER: -5 -3 0 3 5 7

SNACK

WHAT I ATE:

MUFA: CALORIES:

TIME: HUNGER BEFORE: -5 -3 0 3 5 7 | HUNGER AFTER: -5 -3 0 3 5 7

DINNER

WHAT I ATE:

MUFA: CALORIES:

TIME: HUNGER BEFORE: -5 -3 0 3 5 7 | HUNGER AFTER: -5 -3 0 3 5 7

CORE CONFIDENCE:

_____
_____
_____
_____
_____
_____
_____
_____
_____
_____
_____
_____
_____
_____
_____
_____
_____

WORKOUT		
WALKING	Fat Blast Walk _____minutes	Calorie Torch Walk _____minutes
STRENGTH TRAINING	The Belly Routine ____sets____reps	The Metabolism Boost ___sets___reps
HOW I FELT:		

DAY 4

BREAKFAST

WHAT I ATE:

MUFA: CALORIES:

TIME: HUNGER BEFORE: -5 -3 0 3 5 7   HUNGER AFTER: -5 -3 0 3 5 7

LUNCH

WHAT I ATE:

MUFA: CALORIES:

TIME: HUNGER BEFORE: -5 -3 0 3 5 7   HUNGER AFTER: -5 -3 0 3 5 7

SNACK

WHAT I ATE:

MUFA: CALORIES:

TIME: HUNGER BEFORE: -5 -3 0 3 5 7   HUNGER AFTER: -5 -3 0 3 5 7

DINNER

WHAT I ATE:

MUFA: CALORIES:

TIME: HUNGER BEFORE: -5 -3 0 3 5 7   HUNGER AFTER: -5 -3 0 3 5 7

CORE CONFIDENCE:

_____

_____

_____

_____

_____

_____

_____

_____

_____

_____

_____

_____

_____

_____

_____

_____

_____

WORKOUT		
WALKING	Fat Blast Walk _____minutes	Calorie Torch Walk _____minutes
STRENGTH TRAINING	The Belly Routine ____sets____reps	The Metabolism Boost ___sets___reps
HOW I FELT:		

DAY 5

BREAKFAST

WHAT I ATE:

MUFA: CALORIES:

TIME: HUNGER BEFORE: -5 -3 0 3 5 7   HUNGER AFTER: -5 -3 0 3 5 7

LUNCH

WHAT I ATE:

MUFA: CALORIES:

TIME: HUNGER BEFORE: -5 -3 0 3 5 7   HUNGER AFTER: -5 -3 0 3 5 7

SNACK

WHAT I ATE:

MUFA: CALORIES:

TIME: HUNGER BEFORE: -5 -3 0 3 5 7   HUNGER AFTER: -5 -3 0 3 5 7

DINNER

WHAT I ATE:

MUFA: CALORIES:

TIME: HUNGER BEFORE: -5 -3 0 3 5 7   HUNGER AFTER: -5 -3 0 3 5 7

CORE CONFIDENCE:

_____

_____

_____

_____

_____

_____

_____

_____

_____

_____

_____

_____

_____

_____

_____

_____

_____

WORKOUT	
WALKING	Fat Blast Walk _____minutes	Calorie Torch Walk _____minutes
STRENGTH TRAINING	The Belly Routine ____sets____reps	The Metabolism Boost ___sets___reps

HOW I FELT:

DAY 6

BREAKFAST

WHAT I ATE:

MUFA: CALORIES:

TIME: HUNGER BEFORE: -5 -3 0 3 5 7   HUNGER AFTER: -5 -3 0 3 5 7

LUNCH

WHAT I ATE:

MUFA: CALORIES:

TIME: HUNGER BEFORE: -5 -3 0 3 5 7   HUNGER AFTER: -5 -3 0 3 5 7

SNACK

WHAT I ATE:

MUFA: CALORIES:

TIME: HUNGER BEFORE: -5 -3 0 3 5 7   HUNGER AFTER: -5 -3 0 3 5 7

DINNER

WHAT I ATE:

MUFA: CALORIES:

TIME: HUNGER BEFORE: -5 -3 0 3 5 7   HUNGER AFTER: -5 -3 0 3 5 7

CORE CONFIDENCE:

_____

_____

_____

_____

_____

_____

_____

_____

_____

_____

_____

_____

_____

_____

_____

_____

WORKOUT		
WALKING	Fat Blast Walk _____minutes	Calorie Torch Walk _____minutes
STRENGTH TRAINING	The Belly Routine ____sets____reps	The Metabolism Boost ___sets___reps

HOW I FELT:

DAY 7

BREAKFAST

WHAT I ATE:

MUFA: CALORIES:

TIME: HUNGER BEFORE: -5 -3 0 3 5 7   HUNGER AFTER: -5 -3 0 3 5 7

LUNCH

WHAT I ATE:

MUFA: CALORIES:

TIME: HUNGER BEFORE: -5 -3 0 3 5 7   HUNGER AFTER: -5 -3 0 3 5 7

SNACK

WHAT I ATE:

MUFA: CALORIES:

TIME: HUNGER BEFORE: -5 -3 0 3 5 7   HUNGER AFTER: -5 -3 0 3 5 7

DINNER

WHAT I ATE:

MUFA: CALORIES:

TIME: HUNGER BEFORE: -5 -3 0 3 5 7   HUNGER AFTER: -5 -3 0 3 5 7

CORE CONFIDENCE:

_____

_____

_____

_____

_____

_____

_____

_____

_____

_____

_____

_____

_____

_____

_____

_____

_____

WORKOUT		
WALKING	Fat Blast Walk _____minutes	Calorie Torch Walk _____minutes
STRENGTH TRAINING	The Belly Routine ____sets____reps	The Metabolism Boost ___sets___reps

HOW I FELT:

DAY 8

BREAKFAST

WHAT I ATE:

MUFA: CALORIES:

TIME: HUNGER BEFORE: -5 -3 0 3 5 7   HUNGER AFTER: -5 -3 0 3 5 7

LUNCH

WHAT I ATE:

MUFA: CALORIES:

TIME: HUNGER BEFORE: -5 -3 0 3 5 7   HUNGER AFTER: -5 -3 0 3 5 7

SNACK

WHAT I ATE:

MUFA: CALORIES:

TIME: HUNGER BEFORE: -5 -3 0 3 5 7   HUNGER AFTER: -5 -3 0 3 5 7

DINNER

WHAT I ATE:

MUFA: CALORIES:

TIME: HUNGER BEFORE: -5 -3 0 3 5 7   HUNGER AFTER: -5 -3 0 3 5 7

CORE CONFIDENCE:

_____

_____

_____

_____

_____

_____

_____

_____

_____

_____

_____

_____

_____

_____

_____

_____

_____

WORKOUT	
WALKING	Fat Blast Walk _____ minutes	Calorie Torch Walk _____ minutes
STRENGTH TRAINING	The Belly Routine ____ sets ____ reps	The Metabolism Boost ___ sets ___ reps

HOW I FELT:

DAY 9

BREAKFAST

WHAT I ATE:

MUFA: CALORIES:

| TIME: | HUNGER BEFORE: -5 -3 0 3 5 7 | HUNGER AFTER: -5 -3 0 3 5 7 |

LUNCH

WHAT I ATE:

MUFA: CALORIES:

| TIME: | HUNGER BEFORE: -5 -3 0 3 5 7 | HUNGER AFTER: -5 -3 0 3 5 7 |

SNACK

WHAT I ATE:

MUFA: CALORIES:

| TIME: | HUNGER BEFORE: -5 -3 0 3 5 7 | HUNGER AFTER: -5 -3 0 3 5 7 |

DINNER

WHAT I ATE:

MUFA: CALORIES:

| TIME: | HUNGER BEFORE: -5 -3 0 3 5 7 | HUNGER AFTER: -5 -3 0 3 5 7 |

CORE CONFIDENCE:

_____

_____

_____

_____

_____

_____

_____

_____

_____

_____

_____

_____

_____

_____

_____

WORKOUT		
WALKING	Fat Blast Walk _____minutes	Calorie Torch Walk _____minutes
STRENGTH TRAINING	The Belly Routine ____sets____reps	The Metabolism Boost ___sets___reps
HOW I FELT:		

DAY 10

BREAKFAST

WHAT I ATE:

MUFA: CALORIES:

TIME: HUNGER BEFORE: -5 -3 0 3 5 7   HUNGER AFTER: -5 -3 0 3 5 7

LUNCH

WHAT I ATE:

MUFA: CALORIES:

TIME: HUNGER BEFORE: -5 -3 0 3 5 7   HUNGER AFTER: -5 -3 0 3 5 7

SNACK

WHAT I ATE:

MUFA: CALORIES:

TIME: HUNGER BEFORE: -5 -3 0 3 5 7   HUNGER AFTER: -5 -3 0 3 5 7

DINNER

WHAT I ATE:

MUFA: CALORIES:

TIME: HUNGER BEFORE: -5 -3 0 3 5 7   HUNGER AFTER: -5 -3 0 3 5 7

CORE CONFIDENCE:

_____

_____

_____

_____

_____

_____

_____

_____

_____

_____

_____

_____

_____

_____

_____

_____

_____

_____

WORKOUT		
WALKING	Fat Blast Walk _____minutes	Calorie Torch Walk _____minutes
STRENGTH TRAINING	The Belly Routine _____sets_____reps	The Metabolism Boost ___sets___reps
HOW I FELT:		

DAY 11

WHAT I ATE:

MUFA: CALORIES:

TIME: HUNGER BEFORE: -5 -3 0 3 5 7 | HUNGER AFTER: -5 -3 0 3 5 7

LUNCH

WHAT I ATE:

MUFA: CALORIES:

TIME: HUNGER BEFORE: -5 -3 0 3 5 7 | HUNGER AFTER: -5 -3 0 3 5 7

SNACK

WHAT I ATE:

MUFA: CALORIES:

TIME: HUNGER BEFORE: -5 -3 0 3 5 7 | HUNGER AFTER: -5 -3 0 3 5 7

DINNER

WHAT I ATE:

MUFA: CALORIES:

TIME: HUNGER BEFORE: -5 -3 0 3 5 7 | HUNGER AFTER: -5 -3 0 3 5 7

CORE CONFIDENCE:

_____

_____

_____

_____

_____

_____

_____

_____

_____

_____

_____

_____

_____

_____

_____

_____

_____

_____

WORKOUT		
WALKING	Fat Blast Walk _____minutes	Calorie Torch Walk _____minutes
STRENGTH TRAINING	The Belly Routine ____sets____reps	The Metabolism Boost ___sets___reps
HOW I FELT:		

DAY 12

BREAKFAST

WHAT I ATE:

MUFA: CALORIES:

TIME: HUNGER BEFORE: -5 -3 0 3 5 7   HUNGER AFTER: -5 -3 0 3 5 7

LUNCH

WHAT I ATE:

MUFA: CALORIES:

TIME: HUNGER BEFORE: -5 -3 0 3 5 7   HUNGER AFTER: -5 -3 0 3 5 7

SNACK

WHAT I ATE:

MUFA: CALORIES:

TIME: HUNGER BEFORE: -5 -3 0 3 5 7   HUNGER AFTER: -5 -3 0 3 5 7

DINNER

WHAT I ATE:

MUFA: CALORIES:

TIME: HUNGER BEFORE: -5 -3 0 3 5 7   HUNGER AFTER: -5 -3 0 3 5 7

CORE CONFIDENCE:

_____
_____
_____
_____
_____
_____
_____
_____
_____
_____
_____
_____
_____
_____
_____
_____
_____

WORKOUT		
WALKING	Fat Blast Walk _____minutes	Calorie Torch Walk _____minutes
STRENGTH TRAINING	The Belly Routine _____sets_____reps	The Metabolism Boost ___sets___reps

HOW I FELT:

DAY 13

BREAKFAST

WHAT I ATE:

MUFA: CALORIES:

TIME: HUNGER BEFORE: -5 -3 0 3 5 7 | HUNGER AFTER: -5 -3 0 3 5 7

LUNCH

WHAT I ATE:

MUFA: CALORIES:

TIME: HUNGER BEFORE: -5 -3 0 3 5 7 | HUNGER AFTER: -5 -3 0 3 5 7

SNACK

WHAT I ATE:

MUFA: CALORIES:

TIME: HUNGER BEFORE: -5 -3 0 3 5 7 | HUNGER AFTER: -5 -3 0 3 5 7

DINNER

WHAT I ATE:

MUFA: CALORIES:

TIME: HUNGER BEFORE: -5 -3 0 3 5 7 | HUNGER AFTER: -5 -3 0 3 5 7

■ **CORE CONFIDENCE:**

_____

_____

_____

_____

_____

_____

_____

_____

_____

_____

_____

_____

_____

_____

_____

_____

_____

WORKOUT		
WALKING	Fat Blast Walk _____minutes	Calorie Torch Walk _____minutes
STRENGTH TRAINING	The Belly Routine ____sets____reps	The Metabolism Boost ___sets___reps
HOW I FELT:		

DAY 14

BREAKFAST

WHAT I ATE:

MUFA: CALORIES:

| TIME: | HUNGER BEFORE: -5 -3 0 3 5 7 | HUNGER AFTER: -5 -3 0 3 5 7 |

LUNCH

WHAT I ATE:

MUFA: CALORIES:

| TIME: | HUNGER BEFORE: -5 -3 0 3 5 7 | HUNGER AFTER: -5 -3 0 3 5 7 |

SNACK

WHAT I ATE:

MUFA: CALORIES:

| TIME: | HUNGER BEFORE: -5 -3 0 3 5 7 | HUNGER AFTER: -5 -3 0 3 5 7 |

DINNER

WHAT I ATE:

MUFA: CALORIES:

| TIME: | HUNGER BEFORE: -5 -3 0 3 5 7 | HUNGER AFTER: -5 -3 0 3 5 7 |

CORE CONFIDENCE:

_____

_____

_____

_____

_____

_____

_____

_____

_____

_____

_____

_____

_____

WORKOUT	
WALKING	Fat Blast Walk _____minutes	Calorie Torch Walk _____minutes
STRENGTH TRAINING	The Belly Routine ____sets____reps	The Metabolism Boost ___sets___reps

HOW I FELT:

DAY 15

BREAKFAST

WHAT I ATE:

MUFA: CALORIES:

TIME: HUNGER BEFORE: -5 -3 0 3 5 7 | HUNGER AFTER: -5 -3 0 3 5 7

LUNCH

WHAT I ATE:

MUFA: CALORIES:

TIME: HUNGER BEFORE: -5 -3 0 3 5 7 | HUNGER AFTER: -5 -3 0 3 5 7

SNACK

WHAT I ATE:

MUFA: CALORIES:

TIME: HUNGER BEFORE: -5 -3 0 3 5 7 | HUNGER AFTER: -5 -3 0 3 5 7

DINNER

WHAT I ATE:

MUFA: CALORIES:

TIME: HUNGER BEFORE: -5 -3 0 3 5 7 | HUNGER AFTER: -5 -3 0 3 5 7

■ **CORE CONFIDENCE:**

_____

_____

_____

_____

_____

_____

_____

_____

_____

_____

_____

_____

_____

_____

_____

_____

WORKOUT	
WALKING	Fat Blast Walk _____minutes	Calorie Torch Walk _____minutes
STRENGTH TRAINING	The Belly Routine ____sets____reps	The Metabolism Boost ___sets___reps

HOW I FELT:

DAY 16

BREAKFAST

WHAT I ATE:

MUFA: CALORIES:

TIME: | HUNGER BEFORE: -5 -3 0 3 5 7 | HUNGER AFTER: -5 -3 0 3 5 7

LUNCH

WHAT I ATE:

MUFA: CALORIES:

TIME: | HUNGER BEFORE: -5 -3 0 3 5 7 | HUNGER AFTER: -5 -3 0 3 5 7

SNACK

WHAT I ATE:

MUFA: CALORIES:

TIME: | HUNGER BEFORE: -5 -3 0 3 5 7 | HUNGER AFTER: -5 -3 0 3 5 7

DINNER

WHAT I ATE:

MUFA: CALORIES:

TIME: | HUNGER BEFORE: -5 -3 0 3 5 7 | HUNGER AFTER: -5 -3 0 3 5 7

CORE CONFIDENCE:

_____

_____

_____

_____

_____

_____

_____

_____

_____

_____

_____

_____

_____

_____

_____

_____

_____

WORKOUT		
WALKING	Fat Blast Walk _____ minutes	Calorie Torch Walk _____ minutes
STRENGTH TRAINING	The Belly Routine ____sets____reps	The Metabolism Boost ___sets___reps

HOW I FELT:

DAY 17

BREAKFAST

WHAT I ATE:

MUFA: CALORIES:

TIME: HUNGER BEFORE: -5 -3 0 3 5 7 HUNGER AFTER: -5 -3 0 3 5 7

LUNCH

WHAT I ATE:

MUFA: CALORIES:

TIME: HUNGER BEFORE: -5 -3 0 3 5 7 HUNGER AFTER: -5 -3 0 3 5 7

SNACK

WHAT I ATE:

MUFA: CALORIES:

TIME: HUNGER BEFORE: -5 -3 0 3 5 7 HUNGER AFTER: -5 -3 0 3 5 7

DINNER

WHAT I ATE:

MUFA: CALORIES:

TIME: HUNGER BEFORE: -5 -3 0 3 5 7 HUNGER AFTER: -5 -3 0 3 5 7

CORE CONFIDENCE:

WORKOUT		
WALKING	Fat Blast Walk _____minutes	Calorie Torch Walk _____minutes
STRENGTH TRAINING	The Belly Routine ____sets____reps	The Metabolism Boost ___sets___reps
HOW I FELT:		

DAY 18

BREAKFAST

WHAT I ATE:

MUFA: CALORIES:

TIME: HUNGER BEFORE: -5 -3 0 3 5 7   HUNGER AFTER: -5 -3 0 3 5 7

LUNCH

WHAT I ATE:

MUFA: CALORIES:

TIME: HUNGER BEFORE: -5 -3 0 3 5 7   HUNGER AFTER: -5 -3 0 3 5 7

SNACK

WHAT I ATE:

MUFA: CALORIES:

TIME: HUNGER BEFORE: -5 -3 0 3 5 7   HUNGER AFTER: -5 -3 .0 3 5 7

DINNER

WHAT I ATE:

MUFA: CALORIES:

TIME: HUNGER BEFORE: -5 -3 0 3 5 7   HUNGER AFTER: -5 -3 0 3 5 7

CORE CONFIDENCE:

_____

_____

_____

_____

_____

_____

_____

_____

_____

_____

_____

_____

_____

_____

_____

_____

_____

WORKOUT		
WALKING	Fat Blast Walk _____minutes	Calorie Torch Walk _____minutes
STRENGTH TRAINING	The Belly Routine ____sets____reps	The Metabolism Boost ___sets___reps

HOW I FELT:

DAY 19

BREAKFAST

WHAT I ATE:

MUFA: CALORIES:

TIME: HUNGER BEFORE: -5 -3 0 3 5 7 | HUNGER AFTER: -5 -3 0 3 5 7

LUNCH

WHAT I ATE:

MUFA: CALORIES:

TIME: HUNGER BEFORE: -5 -3 0 3 5 7 | HUNGER AFTER: -5 -3 0 3 5 7

SNACK

WHAT I ATE:

MUFA: CALORIES:

TIME: HUNGER BEFORE: -5 -3 0 3 5 7 | HUNGER AFTER: -5 -3 0 3 5 7

DINNER

WHAT I ATE:

MUFA: CALORIES:

TIME: HUNGER BEFORE: -5 -3 0 3 5 7 | HUNGER AFTER: -5 -3 0 3 5 7

■ **CORE CONFIDENCE:**

_____

_____

_____

_____

_____

_____

_____

_____

_____

_____

_____

_____

_____

_____

_____

_____

_____

WORKOUT		
WALKING	Fat Blast Walk _____minutes	Calorie Torch Walk _____minutes
STRENGTH TRAINING	The Belly Routine ____sets____reps	The Metabolism Boost ___sets___reps
HOW I FELT:		

DAY 20

DATE

BREAKFAST

WHAT I ATE:

MUFA: CALORIES:

TIME: HUNGER BEFORE: -5 -3 0 3 5 7   HUNGER AFTER: -5 -3 0 3 5 7

LUNCH

WHAT I ATE:

MUFA: CALORIES:

TIME: HUNGER BEFORE: -5 -3 0 3 5 7   HUNGER AFTER: -5 -3 0 3 5 7

SNACK

WHAT I ATE:

MUFA: CALORIES:

TIME: HUNGER BEFORE: -5 -3 0 3 5 7   HUNGER AFTER: -5 -3 0 3 5 7

DINNER

WHAT I ATE:

MUFA: CALORIES:

TIME: HUNGER BEFORE: -5 -3 0 3 5 7   HUNGER AFTER: -5 -3 0 3 5 7

CORE CONFIDENCE:

_____

_____

_____

_____

_____

_____

_____

_____

_____

_____

_____

_____

_____

_____

_____

_____

WORKOUT		
WALKING	Fat Blast Walk _____minutes	Calorie Torch Walk _____minutes
STRENGTH TRAINING	The Belly Routine ____sets____reps	The Metabolism Boost ___sets___reps
HOW I FELT:		

DAY 21

BREAKFAST

WHAT I ATE:

MUFA: CALORIES:

TIME: HUNGER BEFORE: -5 -3 0 3 5 7   HUNGER AFTER: -5 -3 0 3 5 7

LUNCH

WHAT I ATE:

MUFA: CALORIES:

TIME: HUNGER BEFORE: -5 -3 0 3 5 7   HUNGER AFTER: -5 -3 0 3 5 7

SNACK

WHAT I ATE:

MUFA: CALORIES:

TIME: HUNGER BEFORE: -5 -3 0 3 5 7   HUNGER AFTER: -5 -3 0 3 5 7

DINNER

WHAT I ATE:

MUFA: CALORIES:

TIME: HUNGER BEFORE: -5 -3 0 3 5 7   HUNGER AFTER: -5 -3 0 3 5 7

CORE CONFIDENCE:

_____

_____

_____

_____

_____

_____

_____

_____

_____

_____

_____

_____

_____

_____

_____

_____

WORKOUT		
WALKING	Fat Blast Walk _____minutes	Calorie Torch Walk _____minutes
STRENGTH TRAINING	The Belly Routine ____sets____reps	The Metabolism Boost ___sets___reps
HOW I FELT:		

DAY 22

BREAKFAST

WHAT I ATE:

MUFA: CALORIES:

TIME: HUNGER BEFORE: -5 -3 0 3 5 7   HUNGER AFTER: -5 -3 0 3 5 7

LUNCH

WHAT I ATE:

MUFA: CALORIES:

TIME: HUNGER BEFORE: -5 -3 0 3 5 7   HUNGER AFTER: -5 -3 0 3 5 7

SNACK

WHAT I ATE:

MUFA: CALORIES:

TIME: HUNGER BEFORE: -5 -3 0 3 5 7   HUNGER AFTER: -5 -3 0 3 5 7

DINNER

WHAT I ATE:

MUFA: CALORIES:

TIME: HUNGER BEFORE: -5 -3 0 3 5 7   HUNGER AFTER: -5 -3 0 3 5 7

CORE CONFIDENCE:

WORKOUT

WALKING	Fat Blast Walk _____minutes	Calorie Torch Walk _____minutes
STRENGTH TRAINING	The Belly Routine ____sets____reps	The Metabolism Boost ___sets___reps

HOW I FELT:

DAY 23

BREAKFAST

WHAT I ATE:

MUFA: CALORIES:

TIME: HUNGER BEFORE: -5 -3 0 3 5 7   HUNGER AFTER: -5 -3 0 3 5 7

LUNCH

WHAT I ATE:

MUFA: CALORIES:

TIME: HUNGER BEFORE: -5 -3 0 3 5 7   HUNGER AFTER: -5 -3 0 3 5 7

SNACK

WHAT I ATE:

MUFA: CALORIES:

TIME: HUNGER BEFORE: -5 -3 0 3 5 7   HUNGER AFTER: -5 -3 0 3 5 7

DINNER

WHAT I ATE:

MUFA: CALORIES:

TIME: HUNGER BEFORE: -5 -3 0 3 5 7   HUNGER AFTER: -5 -3 0 3 5 7

CORE CONFIDENCE:

_____

_____

_____

_____

_____

_____

_____

_____

_____

_____

_____

_____

_____

_____

_____

_____

_____

WORKOUT	
WALKING	Fat Blast Walk _____minutes	Calorie Torch Walk _____minutes
STRENGTH TRAINING	The Belly Routine ____sets____reps	The Metabolism Boost ___sets___reps
HOW I FELT:		

DAY 24

BREAKFAST

WHAT I ATE:

MUFA: CALORIES:

TIME: HUNGER BEFORE: -5 -3 0 3 5 7 | HUNGER AFTER: -5 -3 0 3 5 7

LUNCH

WHAT I ATE:

MUFA: CALORIES:

TIME: HUNGER BEFORE: -5 -3 0 3 5 7 | HUNGER AFTER: -5 -3 0 3 5 7

SNACK

WHAT I ATE:

MUFA: CALORIES:

TIME: HUNGER BEFORE: -5 -3 0 3 5 7 | HUNGER AFTER: -5 -3 0 3 5 7

DINNER

WHAT I ATE:

MUFA: CALORIES:

TIME: HUNGER BEFORE: -5 -3 0 3 5 7 | HUNGER AFTER: -5 -3 0 3 5 7

CORE CONFIDENCE:

_____

_____

_____

_____

_____

_____

_____

_____

_____

_____

_____

_____

_____

_____

_____

_____

_____

WORKOUT	
WALKING	Fat Blast Walk _____minutes	Calorie Torch Walk _____minutes
STRENGTH TRAINING	The Belly Routine ____sets____reps	The Metabolism Boost ___sets___reps
HOW I FELT:		

DAY 25

BREAKFAST

WHAT I ATE:

MUFA: CALORIES:

| TIME: | HUNGER BEFORE: -5 -3 0 3 5 7 | HUNGER AFTER: -5 -3 0 3 5 7 |

LUNCH

WHAT I ATE:

MUFA: CALORIES:

| TIME: | HUNGER BEFORE: -5 -3 0 3 5 7 | HUNGER AFTER: -5 -3 0 3 5 7 |

SNACK

WHAT I ATE:

MUFA: CALORIES:

| TIME: | HUNGER BEFORE: -5 -3 0 3 5 7 | HUNGER AFTER: -5 -3 0 3 5 7 |

DINNER

WHAT I ATE:

MUFA: CALORIES:

| TIME: | HUNGER BEFORE: -5 -3 0 3 5 7 | HUNGER AFTER: -5 -3 0 3 5 7 |

▨ CORE CONFIDENCE:

_____

_____

_____

_____

_____

_____

_____

_____

_____

_____

_____

_____

_____

_____

_____

_____

_____

WORKOUT	
WALKING	Fat Blast Walk _____minutes	Calorie Torch Walk _____minutes
STRENGTH TRAINING	The Belly Routine ____sets____reps	The Metabolism Boost ___sets___reps
HOW I FELT:	

DAY 26

BREAKFAST

WHAT I ATE:

MUFA: CALORIES:

TIME: HUNGER BEFORE: -5 -3 0 3 5 7 | HUNGER AFTER: -5 -3 0 3 5 7

LUNCH

WHAT I ATE:

MUFA: CALORIES:

TIME: HUNGER BEFORE: -5 -3 0 3 5 7 | HUNGER AFTER: -5 -3 0 3 5 7

SNACK

WHAT I ATE:

MUFA: CALORIES:

TIME: HUNGER BEFORE: -5 -3 0 3 5 7 | HUNGER AFTER: -5 -3 0 3 5 7

DINNER

WHAT I ATE:

MUFA: CALORIES:

TIME: HUNGER BEFORE: -5 -3 0 3 5 7 | HUNGER AFTER: -5 -3 0 3 5 7

■ CORE CONFIDENCE:

_____

_____

_____

_____

_____

_____

_____

_____

_____

_____

_____

_____

_____

_____

_____

_____

_____

WORKOUT	
WALKING	Fat Blast Walk _____minutes	Calorie Torch Walk _____minutes
STRENGTH TRAINING	The Belly Routine ____sets____reps	The Metabolism Boost ___sets___reps

HOW I FELT:

DAY 27

BREAKFAST

WHAT I ATE:

MUFA: CALORIES:

TIME: HUNGER BEFORE: -5 -3 0 3 5 7 | HUNGER AFTER: -5 -3 0 3 5 7

LUNCH

WHAT I ATE:

MUFA: CALORIES:

TIME: HUNGER BEFORE: -5 -3 0 3 5 7 | HUNGER AFTER: -5 -3 0 3 5 7

SNACK

WHAT I ATE:

MUFA: CALORIES:

TIME: HUNGER BEFORE: -5 -3 0 3 5 7 | HUNGER AFTER: -5 -3 0 3 5 7

DINNER

WHAT I ATE:

MUFA: CALORIES:

TIME: HUNGER BEFORE: -5 -3 0 3 5 7 | HUNGER AFTER: -5 -3 0 3 5 7

CORE CONFIDENCE:

_____

_____

_____

_____

_____

_____

_____

_____

_____

_____

_____

_____

_____

_____

WORKOUT		
WALKING	Fat Blast Walk _____ minutes	Calorie Torch Walk _____ minutes
STRENGTH TRAINING	The Belly Routine ____ sets ____ reps	The Metabolism Boost ___ sets ___ reps

HOW I FELT:

DAY 28

BREAKFAST

WHAT I ATE:

MUFA: CALORIES:

TIME: HUNGER BEFORE: -5 -3 0 3 5 7   HUNGER AFTER: -5 -3 0 3 5 7

LUNCH

WHAT I ATE:

MUFA: CALORIES:

TIME: HUNGER BEFORE: -5 -3 0 3 5 7   HUNGER AFTER: -5 -3 0 3 5 7

SNACK

WHAT I ATE:

MUFA: CALORIES:

TIME: HUNGER BEFORE: -5 -3 0 3 5 7   HUNGER AFTER: -5 -3 0 3 5 7

DINNER

WHAT I ATE:

MUFA: CALORIES:

TIME: HUNGER BEFORE: -5 -3 0 3 5 7   HUNGER AFTER: -5 -3 0 3 5 7

CORE CONFIDENCE:

_____

_____

_____

_____

_____

_____

_____

_____

_____

_____

_____

_____

_____

_____

_____

_____

WORKOUT

WALKING	Fat Blast Walk _____minutes	Calorie Torch Walk _____minutes
STRENGTH TRAINING	The Belly Routine ____sets____reps	The Metabolism Boost ___sets___reps

HOW I FELT: